Dr. Vinod Verma

Losing Weight

with
Ayurveda and Yoga

Dr. Vinod Verma

Losing Weight
with
Ayurveda and Yoga

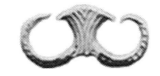

Gayatri Books International

This book is not for sick people or persons with over-weight due to some disease. This is meant for normal healthy persons who have all the basic functions of their body in order. The information provided in this book is not intended to replace the services of a physician. Suggestions for losing weight for better appearance with Ayurvedic methods are given in this book for the self-help and education. The author and the publisher are in no way responsible for any medical claims regarding the material presented in this book. For using methods and remedies provided in this book at commercial level requires the prior permission from the author. For more information, write to the author directly.

© Dr. Vinod Verma 2005 First published in German

Present edition: 2007

Present edition is published by Gayatri Books International, Himalayan Centre, Village Astal, Dunda, Uttarkashi-249151 (Uttarakhanda), India. Any legal matters will be handled in the jurisdiction of this address.

Translation rights are held by the author. Write to her at drvinodverma@dataone.in or ayurvedavv@yahoo.com, or through the publisher at gayatribooks@yahoo.de.

Visit Dr. Vinod Verma at www.ayurvedavv.com to find out about her other publications and other activities like seminars, lectures, consultations etc. Look for more information on the last pages of the book.

Editor: Mahendra Kulasrestha

Cover design: Vanaja Vishal

Book design: Mohit Joshi

ISBN: 81-901722-6-3

Dedicated to the Ayurvedic and yogic sages who provided us the multidimensional wisdom beyond space and time.

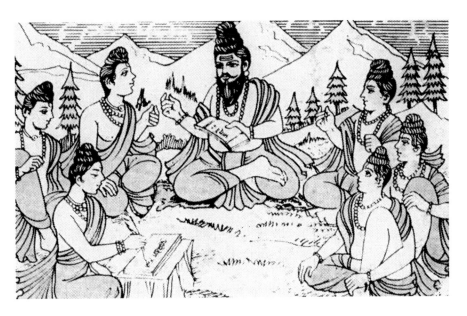

Preface

There are hundreds of books and diets in this world on how to lose weight, then why another book? What is the need of losing weight with Ayurveda? I find that I should answer these two questions before I offer you convenient and healthy Ayurvedic methods to lose as well as to maintain the right weight.

Every now and then, there is a big talk about a new regimen to lose weight with an '*easy and quick method*'. Recently a friend from Germany wrote to me that he had learnt a wonderful regimen to lose weight from his American friends. According to this method, you are not supposed to eat any animal fat but can eat all the vegetables and fruits. Thus, milk, cheese, butter, yoghurt, etc., (also meat and its products for non-vegetarians) should not be taken. The vegetables can be cooked in a very tiny amount of plant fat. I was meeting this friend, who is around fifty, after several months. He had managed to lose his extra 6 kilos but he looked 10 years older and his usual radiating complexion had vanished. His complexion looked dull and ash-coloured. People around him asked him whether he was unwell.

My idea to write this book is to save people from harming themselves due to this kind of ignorance. Ayurveda is a science of life based upon balance and harmony. For example, the above-described regimens will be strictly forbidden in Ayurveda. Due to lack of animal fat and fat in general, the body will acquire an imbalance of vata (ether and air elements). This imbalance will give rise to one or more of the following— rough skin, bad complexion, restlessness, irritation and sleep disorders. Besides these, if you fill yourself more with vegetables and fruits, your pitta (the fire element) will also be disturbed. There will be enhanced excrements and the balance between *mala* (all that body throws out in the form of stool, urine, sweat, etc.) and rasa (all that body assimilates from food) is lost. Due to that, one loses not only weight but also the ojas (immunity and vitality) from the body. Thus, the whole system is disturbed; one loses beauty and charm and acquires haggard looks.

There are similar kinds of problems which people face with other diets as most of these diets are based on leaving out one particular component of the food like proteins, fat or carbohydrates. Excessive intake of proteins, less fat and almost no carbohydrates is a very effective and popular method of losing weight these days but again it is an imbalanced diet and many people suffer from it as their system is not used to excess of proteins with less fat and no carbohydrates.

This explanation answers both the above questions about the purpose of writing this book.

Loss of excessive weight should rejuvenate you and you should acquire more strength. Whether it is prevention or curing ailments or losing or gaining weight, the fundamentals of Ayurveda are based upon maintaining equilibrium of the body. Thus, due to this principle, Ayurveda teaches us to deal with caution and wisdom.

Awareness of the factors that enhance weight is extremely important. Mostly people relate to the theme of balancing weight exclusively with food and exercise. There are several other factors which contribute to enhance body weight and their awareness can benefit for losing and balancing weight. Lifestyle errors that contribute to gain weight are also an important part of this book.

To be able to lose weight on specific parts of the body to shape and trim is the wish of many. Special guidance with Ayurvedic yoga is provided for this purpose.

Ayurveda not only lays emphasis on the equilibrium of the body but also the balance of the three dimensions of mind is extremely important for holistic health. It is important to be aware of the psychological factors that lead to put on extra weight in many cases. It is a vikara or the error of the mind when people eat excessively out of greed. The vikara of the mind may be caused by frustration. Frustration is generally due to lack of wisdom about life and the cosmos. The psychological factors that contribute to weight enhancing are also discussed in the book. They will help you to be aware and not to find solutions to your problems through excessive eating. Equilibrium of the activities of the mind should be maintained with sattva (purity and stillness of mind).

During weight loss, the body decreases in volume and has to reorganise itself in terms of the element space. I have taken care to give you solutions for not getting loose skin, stretch marks or tissue drainage in the process of losing weight.

All this inter-related research and compilation of various Ayurvedic practices along with yogic and other exercises makes this book different from other existing books and methods. Losing weight should mean rejuvenating by shedding the un-needed excessive weight you were carrying with you as a burden.

I have explained every step in this book in such a way that for using this book, you do not require any prior knowledge of Ayurveda. Wherever the terminology of Ayurveda is used, I have given explanations.

I hope that this research based on the ancient wisdom of Ayurveda will provide many people with a solution to their long existing problems about imbalance of body weight and related health problems.

Dr. V. Verma   June 2004

www.ayurvedavv.com

drvinodverma@dataone.in

Ayurvedavv@yahoo.com

Acknowledgements

It is not possible for me to write any book without the help of my Ayurvedic Guru Professor Priya Vrat Sharma. He imparts his tremendous wisdom with generosity. I express my profound gratitude to him.

I acknowledge my gratitude to Mahendra Kulasrestha for a very careful editing and for his valuable suggestions.

I am grateful to Gauree Gayatri, who was once again a wonderful model with patience and indulgence.

I am thankful to the Institute of National Museum for providing some of the art works.

I am indebted to Mohit Joshi for his technical assistance and for extending his generous help in any time of need.

Contents

Section III

Appendix

Ancient texts of Ayurveda on problems of overweight

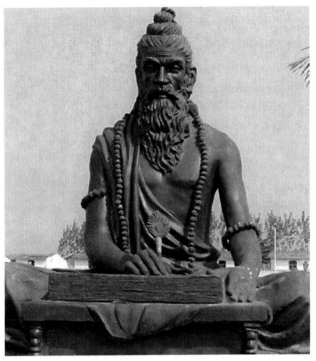

The great sage Charaka wrote 2600 years ago*:

Over-weight persons have eight factors that harm them:

i)   shortening of life span

ii)   hampered movements

iii)   difficulty in sexual intercourse

iv)   debility

v)   foul smell

vi)   over-sweating

vii)   too much hunger and

viii) excessive thirst

---

* Cited from the Caraka Samhita, translation by P. V. Sharma, 1981, Chaukhamba
Orientalia, Varanasi.

Causes

Obesity is caused due to

- ☐ over-saturation,
- ☐ intake of heavy, sweet, cold and fatty diet,
- ☐ indulgence in day sleep,
- ☐ exhilaration,
- ☐ lack of mental work and
- ☐ genetic defects.

Effects

- ☐ In an obese person, there is excess of fat as compared to the other dhatus, therefore the life span is shortened.
- ☐ Because of laxity, softness and heaviness of fat, the movements are hampered.
- ☐ Due to non-abundance of the sexual excretion and their hindered passage due to fat, there is difficulty in sexual activities.
- ☐ Due to the imbalance of dhatus, there is debility.
- ☐ Foul smell is due to vitiation in the quality of fat and due to sweating.
- ☐ Kapha has oozing nature, abundance, heaviness and intolerance to physical exercise and its association with medas (adipose tissue) gives rise to over-sweating.
- ☐ Because of intensified agni, and abundance of vayu (wind) in the belly, there is excessive hunger and thirst.

Charaka Samhita
600 BC

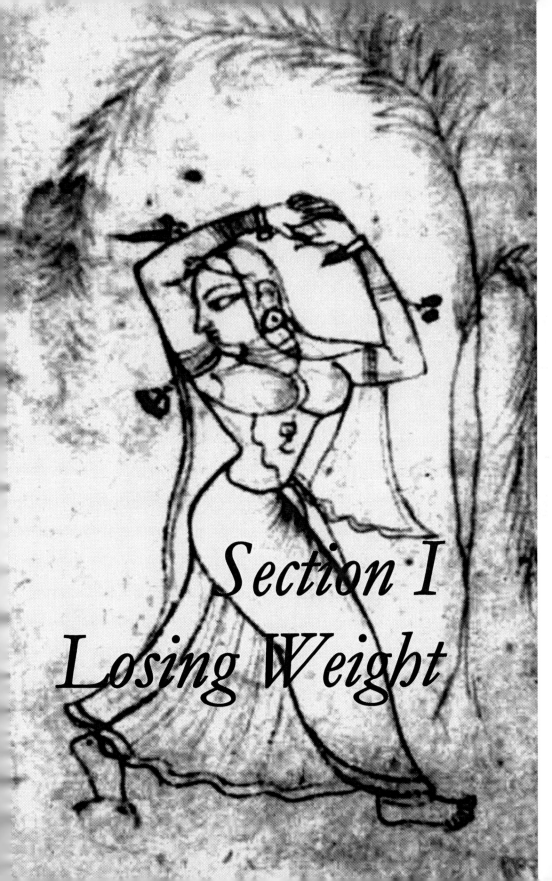

Section I
Losing Weight

1

The Weight-enhancing Factors and How to Deal with Them

Before dealing with the principal theme, let us see what overweight is. I observe people with overweight and de-shaped bodies in the cities in comparison to the people of my village in the mountains. There are no paunches and heavy waistlines up there. What is interesting is that the city people have always some explanation for their extra kilos. If I compare the two folks I come across, the plausible explanations are— lack of movements compared to the intake of food, undisciplined lifestyle and intake of junk food.

The overweight should be seen in terms of the shape of your body and the ease of your mobility. Overweight of even a few kilos makes your body-shape disproportionate and makes you feel heavy, lethargic and breathless. Thus, more than the extra kilos on the scale, you should look at the shape of your body and your agility to judge the overweight. Since even a little over-weight lessens agility, one falls into a vicious cycle and goes on gaining weight due to lethargy caused by the excess weight. To get out of this cycle, one needs strong determination to remain active

It is extremely important to be aware of the major factors that contribute to enhance weight. If you are young and slightly overweight, you may be able to solve your excess weight problem simply by avoiding these factors. I have compiled below a list of diverse factors which are bulk-promoting and have given suggestions for dealing with them.

1. Foods grown with fertilizers
2. Sprayed, processed and preserved foods
3. Limiting oneself in space

4. Going to bed immediately after dinner or eating snacks between dinner and going to bed

5. Excessive sleep

6. Imbalanced diet according to Ayurvedic principles

7. Lack of factor-S in nutrition

8. Nutrition not according to space and time

9. Disturbed balance of rasa and mala

10. Defective and prolonged sitting postures

11. A state of mind that predominates in tamas (greed, laziness and languor)

12. End of the pitta phase of one's life and beginning of middle age

Let us now examine these factors one by one in detail and find ways to combat them.

1. Foods grown with fertilizers

Use of the chemical fertilizers changes the basic equilibrium of the food products. When we consume them, we take excess of nitrates in food product that cause an imbalance of vata and pitta in the body. Pitta is responsible for the digestive fire or agni of the body and thus, it disturbs the energy system of the body. Vata is responsible for the distribution of energy and its disturbance along with pitta imbalances the thermodynamic system of the body. The symptoms are excessive thirst, imbalanced appetite, excessive intake of food and bloating. The body holds water and gradually puts on weight.

Solution: Eat organically grown foods as far as possible.

2. Sprayed, processed and preserved foods

These foods have similar effect as described above. Pesticides and other chemicals disturb the digestive fire of the body and enhance the intake of liquids. They make the body flabby. Processed and preserved foods have certain amount of chemicals in the form of preservatives and colours etc. which do not belong to the natural food and are contrary to the nature of the biological systems. They usually imbalance vata and pitta and make the blood impure. This later gradually affects the water-system of the body (vata and kapha). If these foods are taken in excess, they ultimately disturb all the three energies of the body and cause various ailments besides making the body heavy and flabby.

The preserved and processed foods grown with chemical fertilizers and pesticides are lacking in prana energy or the living element of the cosmos and thus, they do not enrich the body's energy and provide internal satisfaction one should feel after having eaten. I have done no scientific study on this theme as yet, but my general observation is that this kind of food does not appease the hunger along with mental satisfaction and fulfilment, as compared to the organically grown fresh food. Therefore, one tends to eat more than required (see also the description of S- Factor in number 7). Thus, besides the side-effects of the chemicals, there is an added effect of putting on weight with the consumption of these foodstuffs which are anti-nature and are lacking in prana.

Solution: Eat organically grown foods as far as possible. If the vegetables are sprayed, wash them several times with water and soak them in water. Finally, wash them with hot water to get rid of the poisons as much as possible. Eat fresh foods and never consume foods which are prepared several hours before consumption. Never buy readymade food, they usually have preservatives.

3. Limiting oneself in space*

In Ayurveda, the three energies which are responsible for all the physical and mental functions of the body are constituted of five elements. Vata is from ether (space) and air, pitta is from fire and kapha is from water and earth. Generally, the space element of vata is ignored in modern books on Ayurveda. It is important in the present context, as merely losing calories

* For more details on this theme, see Chapter 7 of this section.

by exercise is not the only consideration for weight-balancing from the Ayurvedic point of view. In other words, you should not limit yourself to narrow spaces like homes and offices. There are many people, specially women, who say that they have enough physical exercise at home with children and other household chores. From Ayurvedic point of view, the body is not a mechanical system and the element of space is very important for balancing the body's dynamism.

Solution: Make it a point to go for a walk at least once a day. You should do this specially if your daily activities are limited to indoors.

4. Going to bed immediately after dinner or eating snacks between dinner and going to bed

Many people think that it is healthy to eat early dinner. However, if they go to bed late, they feel hungry and eat snacks between dinner and going to bed. This habit is not only bulk-promoting but is also bad for your general health. Your body is working hard to digest the food you have eaten. Before going to bed, the active process of digestion should be over and the body should be prepared for sleep. The energy channels or srotas of your body gradually close with the nightfall. Eating shortly before going to bed, you force your digestive system with workload when it is already in a state of partial rest. This leads to many stomach ailments besides promoting weight.

Solution: Decide the time of your dinner not by clock but according to your sleeping habits. You should have your dinner at least two hours before going to bed. Going for walk after dinner is highly recommended. Leave a gap of 12 hours between your dinner and breakfast.

5. Excessive sleep

Babies and small children need lots of sleep whereas adults need a maximum of eight hours sleep. For a healthy adult, I recommend not more than seven hours of sleep with the exception of some special circumstances like being sick or after excessive work or travelling. Persons with kapha energy dominance like to sleep a lot. They tend to lose balance in this respect and if given an opportunity, they would love to use their spare time lazing around and sleeping. More sleep than required not only makes you put on weight but also makes you dull and slow. Sleep is one of the major bulk-promoting factors.

Solution: Be very disciplined in your sleeping hours. If you feel that you have an uncontrollable urge to sleep a lot or you feel very drowsy after meals or you oversleep unless you put an alarm, you need to check on your state of health. Feeling drowsy after meals signifies that your digestive functions are not all right. Sleeping until late in the morning and not feeling like getting up signifies an imbalance of kapha energy. You need to promote the digestive fire in both the cases. Include ginger, garlic, ajwain, cumin, pepper and long pepper in your meals. Take lemon and ginger juice in water everyday. Do physical exercises regularly. Lastly, make an effort to limit your sleep to appropriate hours. These are the kapha energy balancing measures and with these you will come out of the vicious cycle of kapha imbalance and sleeping excessively due to it.

6. Imbalanced diet according to Ayurvedic principles

Taking diet that predominates in kapha and vata and consuming nutrition which is deficient in rasas that have the fire element (pitta) leads to promoting bulk. In other words, the three principal energies of the body get out of balance due to imbalanced diet. Kapha is the energy of water and earth which are the two heavy elements; vata is from air and space which are everywhere in the body and signify volume, whereas pitta is the balancing factor between the two by regulating the thermodynamics of the body.

Solution: Follow the recipes given in this book not only for losing weight but also for balancing the thermodynamics of your body. See the Appendix for some more details about the Ayurvedic nature of food products. To understand and follow the Ayurvedic nutrition principles and recipes based upon them, consult my book⁻ *Ayurvedic Food Culture and Recipes* (see appendix for reference).

7. Lack of S-factor in nutrition

S represents satisfaction in this case. Food appeases our hunger, nourishes us and besides that, it also provides us with some subtle energy. I call it 'the living element or prana in food'. Depending upon where the food is grown and how it is grown and interaction of the growing plants with other living bodies of nature, as well as with rain, sun, wind and other environmental factors; the food has more or less subtle energy or element of prana in it. Besides that, the use of various seeds as spices enriches the food in subtle energy. Seeds have potentials in them to grow into plants and they have abundance of subtle energy or prana energy. Food provides us nourishment and appeases hunger, whereas the prana energy in food gives us a subtle energy and a sense of satisfaction. If prana energy* is missing from the food we consume, we do not feel 'satisfied' or enriched with energy and go on eating in large quantities. This leads to over-weight in due course of time.

Solution: It is very important to buy good quality food, enrich it with herbs and spices and prepare it with great love to enhance the S-factor. You should use a large variety of products and even if you do not use too many spices, think of adding sesame seeds, pumpkin, sunflower or other similar seeds into your salads or other dishes to enhance the S-factor in your food.

8. Nutrition not according to space and time

Kala (the time) and desha (the space) are two very important factors in Ayurvedic food culture. Time is in terms of our age, time of the day and

---

* For more details of prana in food, consult my book, *Ayurvedic Food Culture and Recipes.*

time of the year. Space is in terms of geographical location and environment. For an Ayurvedic lifestyle, one should live according to desha and kala. For example, if you live in the tropical regions of the globe, the food is different whereas in cold countries, the nutrition has to be changed. In hot climate, you need more salt and if you move to a colder part of the globe and continue to consume highly salty and spicy diet, you will retain water and enhance your weight. In cold countries, you need a diet with a little more fat and proteins as compared to the hot countries. If you eat the same diet in hot countries, you will gain weight as due to heat, the thermodynamic system of the body works in a different manner.

You need to change your nutrition according to time of the day and year, and your age. If you eat the same diet in your youth in quality and quantity as you ate during childhood, you may gain weight. Similarly, when you step into middle age from youth, which is predominant in vata and do not change your diet accordingly, you may gain few extra kilos that you may find hard to get rid of.

Solution: Make every effort to make your nutrition according to desha and kala. If you happen to move from one place to another change you diet and eat the way people of that region eat. Change your diet according to season, specify your nutrition with the day and eat according to your age. I have given below a table suggesting some foods and precautions according to age. The tables to show the Ayurvedic nature of different foods are given in the Appendix.

Table to show the predominance of various energies in the three different phases of life, and suggested foods and precautions

Phase of life	Predominant energy	Suggested foods	Precautions
Childhood	Kapha	Sweet and fatty foods should be balanced with ginger, garlic cumin, ajwain. Saffron, pepper, basil, etc. Vegetable or chicken soups should be taken.	Take candy sugar instead of normal sugar; avoid too many sweet and fat containing foods.
Youth	Pitta	The above-described spices should be taken in a moderate quantity, enhance the intake of liquids, eat plenty of salads and fruits, avoid pork and eggs and take fish and mutton	Avoid dill seeds, garlic, and saffron in summer. Treat skin eruptions with wormwood tea and include plenty of bitter tasting foods in your menu.
Middle age and old age	Vata	Take vata-balancing substances like fenugreek, cumin, ajwain, saffron and ginger. Begin to eat less in quantity and stick to early and light dinners but warm. Decrease the intake of salt.	Get used to this phase of life by reducing the intake of food and absolutely refraining from over-eating, even in parties. Take very little salt for dinner. Drink hot water boiled with cardamom few times a day.

9. Disturbed balance of rasa and mala

All what we consume in the body is split into rasa (the essence of the food that body absorbs) and mala (the elements body does not absorb and are thrown out in the form of excrements). In some cases, the balance between rasa and mala is lost. The mala is thrown out in a disproportionate way. If you have less mala in proportion to what you eat, you will put on weight. On the contrary, if the mala is in excess and is in disproportionate to the rasa, you will lose weight. If the problem of imbalance persists, one becomes underweight.

Solution: To create a balance between rasa and mala, take a treatment of trifala with water for two weeks (see chapter 4 of this section). Make sure that you have good evacuation and no partial constipation. Drink a glass of hot water upon getting up in the morning and do some yogic exercises or take a walk. This promotes stool. Get into the habit of going to the toilet twice a day. Drink some hot water half an hour before dinner and make an effort to go to the toilet.

10. Defective and prolonged sitting postures

Prolonged sitting and with odd body positions may make you gain weight on some specific parts of your body. Sitting long hours to do desk work and working with computer generally leads to fat accumulation around the abdomen. Some women tend to gain weight on thighs and hips.

Defective postures lead to vata vitiation and that in turn may become one of the factors to gain weight.

Solution: Always break long sitting postures with some movements. Do some stretching exercises in between. Make sure that you walk a little after lunch and compensate for lack of movements during the weekends and holidays.

11. A state of mind that predominates in tamas (greed or lobha, laziness and languor)

Thinking process undergoes three basic types of modification— rajas, tamas and sattva. Rajas is the active principle, tamas is the inactive principle that also includes those modifications of mind that hinder development of mind and sattva is inner peace and stillness. Sattva is the balancing factor for rajas and tamas which are generally predominant in modern day life. Feelings like anger, greed, excessive attachment, laziness and languor are in the category of tamas as they hinder the mental development of a person.

Lobha or greed is the desire to have more and more to oneself. In the present context of overweight, it has two aspects. Excessive intake of food becomes the cause of over-weight and ailments. Many people tend to consume good food in large quantities and more than their system can handle. They have access to fine tasting foods and for the pleasure of the tongue, they eat more than needed. The second aspect of lobha is that there are people who are busy accumulating wealth and they find that they do not have time to cook and eat food that is fresh, balanced and ojas (immunity and vitality) promoting. Therefore they eat anti-health food that lowers their ojas and also makes them over-weight.

Solutions: Keep a control on your mind and never overeat. If the food is extremely appeasing for your senses, eat slowly and enjoy more but keep a vigil on yourself never to eat in excess. To attain control over your mind, do some concentration and meditative practices.

12. End of the pitta phase of one's life and beginning of the middle age

According to Ayurveda, the childhood is predominant in kapha whereas youth is pitta dominant. Old age dominates in vata (see the table given above). At the end of the prime of youth, between 45-50 years of age, we slowly step into middle age and get vata energy in predominance. That means the thermodynamic system of the body changes with age. Lesser pitta energy signifies lesser digestive fire. Therefore, you need to change your food habits according to age. The nutrition, which is normally converted into heat energy during the youth, begins to accumulate in the body at this age. In addition to that, with a lessened energy as compared to youth, most people have relatively lesser mobility and activity at this age. Therefore, all this results in enhancing weight.

Solution: You need to change your food habits with age. You should also keep up with some physical activity in a very regular manner. Eat feast meals rarely and never overeat. Eat a variety of things in your meal and lay emphasis on mixed vegetables, mixed fruit salads, use of a variety of spices as has been described in the recipes in the next chapter. Follow strictly the eight golden principles of Ayurveda (see Chapter 2 of Section II). When we are young, the body takes irregularities and excesses easily and recovers back to prakriti (state of health). However, at the end of youth, the ojas of the body decline and we need to pay more attention. In brief, eat regular meals with a variety of ingredients but never over-eat. Exercise and intake of rasayanas will help keep the vigour and will save you from putting on weight.

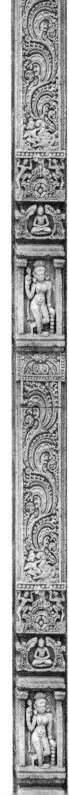

2

Seven-week Nutrition Programme

Before you begin your diet plan, it is essential to prepare yourself for it from Ayurvedic point of view. You need to do simply some purification of the body to gain balance of the body's agni or digestive fire. The diet given in this book is different from your usual notion of the diet to reduce weight. Normally people associate with diet the meals, which are not appetizing and pleasurable. There is nothing like it in the Ayurvedic diet plan I have made for you. They are good and tasty vegetarian meals. Each meal has a dessert. This diet will not only help you to shed your extra kilos but it will also make you feel dynamic and rejuvenated.

Preparing the body for the special diet

The principal preparation is to balance the body's digestive fire called agni in Ayurveda. Agni is a part of the pitta energy of the body and it is important to bring it in equilibrium. With balanced agni, your hunger, thirst, digestion and assimilation of the food regains an equilibrium. For example, some people put on weight because they feel excessively and frequently hungry. They are disturbed with the hunger and are compelled to eat. In fact, their agni is disturbed and they get false hunger alarms. There are others who put on weight because they have excess of agni or digestive fire and consume large quantities of food. It makes sense that before you begin the seven-week diet programme, you balance the thermodynamics of your body for obtaining optimum results.

The major step to balance the pitta energy as well as agni is done with purgation. However, before purgation, body has to be prepared for this process of purification.

Purgation for balancing pitta

Purgation is done by taking purgative substances in the evening, before going to bed. Pay attention to the following before you take a purgative.

- ☐ You should not be ill or suffering from fatigue.
- ☐ Prepare your body for about 10 days beforehand with massage, fomentation and rest.
- ☐ Bring your mind to rest.
- ☐ Decrease your stomach's capacity and demand by exercising self-control. Make an effort to eat only two third of stomach full. Do not eat anything between meals and be strict about it.

Preparation for purgation

Purgation purifies the body in general and specifically, it purifies the liver and other digestive glands. For any kind of purification in Ayurveda, the body has to be prepared so that the impurities are loosened and come out with facility. For this purpose, make a relaxation programme for about ten days.

Application of oil and fomentation*: Apply some warm oil on your body and massage properly on your own or get yourself massaged. After the oil application, do some fomentation by sitting in a hot bath with some essential oils. Use oils of rose, jasmine, sandalwood, eucalyptus or citronella. There are combinations of such oils available in the market for bath. Sit in the bath until you begin to sweat.

Come out of the bath, put on your bathrobe and get into bed to take rest. Your body will continue to sweat. Drink ginger tea, which should be pre-prepared and kept in a thermos near your bed. This will compensate for the loss of fluid from your body and help the process of fomentation.

---

* For details of oil saturation self-massage and fomentation, refer to my book *Programming Your Life With Ayurveda*.

Make sure that there is no air draft while you are bathing or doing fomentation.

During the ten days of relaxation, repeat this process twice.

Choice and dose of the purgative

Every country has its purgatives which are generally used to cure constipation. However, you need a stronger dose (two to three times) than the one taken to cure constipation. The purgative could be from a single plant or mixture of several plants.

Powdered leaves of Sanaye (*Cassia augustifolia*) is a very good purgative for purification. Take about 1 teaspoon of this powder with warm water before going to bed.

Alternatively, the pulp of amaltas (*Cassia fistula*) can be taken. Take out the pulp from about 12-13 cm (about 5 inches) of the bean stock. Beans are between 30 cm (1 foot) to 60 cm (2 feet) long. Boil the pulp in a little water. Mash it properly and filter it through a strainer. Drink it at night before going to bed.

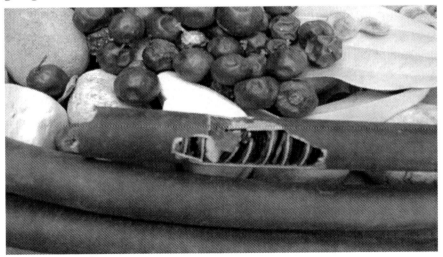

Reaction: Purgatives are taken in the evening before going to bed. They work inside you during the night and depending on your state of health, you may have stomach-ache or flatus before you get loose motions. The reaction time naturally varies from one individual to another. Some of you may feel a strong urge to go to the toilet during the early hours of the morning; others will need some time after getting up and have to drink something before the reaction begins. It is not important when the purging begins. What matters is that it occurs several times until there is only water coming out. If you do not purge properly and you have only one or two motions, repeat the process with a higher dose.

After purgation: Take light liquid meals like soups, rice and easily digestible vegetables like zucchini, pumpkin, carrots, turnips etc. Eat only cooked food. Take some rest and avoid doing any physical labour for two days.

Seven-week Diet Plan

I will give you below seven different diet plans. Each plan has to be repeated after seven days. Keep repeating this diet for seven weeks. I have given all the preparation methods, recipes and other details on the following pages.

This diet with low fat contents is very tasty. There is no suffering involved as the preparations are of high quality and with spices and there is a dessert with each meal. According to Ayurvedic principles, one must close the stomach with sweet. The diet plan is prepared on the principles of Ayurveda. Each meal has diverse rasas or essential elements from varied tastes. The meals will give you a sense of satisfaction and will not leave you frustrated like the most diets.

The principle recipes of the main dishes are given after the diet plan. They are referred to by names or numbers in the plan.

Day 1

Morning drink: Many people drink something upon getting up. It is generally a warm drink taken before breakfast. In India, people generally drink either tea or coffee with milk and sugar. You can do that but gradually try to reduce the quantity of sugar in your drink. I highly recommend an Eleven-spice rejuvenating drink that I have put together. This will give you energy for the day and will balance the body fire (pitta). In addition to that, this drink does not need sugar as it has two ingredients, which are naturally sweet.

Eleven-spice Rejuvenating and Anti-fatigue tea

This tea is a rasayana or a rejuvenating tea. It is better to make this tea mixture in bulk for everyday use.

Ingredients:

Coriander seeds	50 gm (2 ounce)
Dried ginger	50 gm (2 ounce)
Liquorice	50 gm (2 ounce)
Fennel	50 gm (2 ounce)
Cardamom seeds	25 gm (1 ounce)
Big cardamom seeds	25 gm (1 ounce)
Dried basil leaves (*Tulsi*)	25 gm (1 ounce)
Long pepper*	25 gm (1 ounce)
Black pepper	25 gm (1 ounce)
Clove	25 gm (1 ounce)
Cinnamon	25 gm (1 ounce)

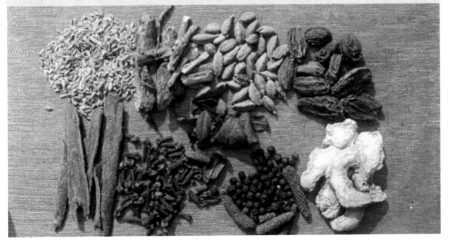

Clean and powder all these ingredients with the electric grinder. Mix the powder well and pass it through a strainer to make sure that there are no big pieces left. Grind once again the contents you obtain on the strainer. Make sure to mix well the final powder you have obtained. Store this powder in a tightly closed dried jar. Take out a small amount for everyday use.

Make the tea by using ½ teaspoon of this powder in ½ litre (2½ cup) of water. Boil the water on low fire for about three minutes with a lid on. Let the tea rest as such for three more minutes before serving.

Note: Those of you who are used to taking black tea or coffee can try the following recipe. Add a teaspoon of black tea (granular black tea like the English Breakfast Tea) in the above preparation after having boiled the rejuvenation mixture for three minutes. Let the black tea boil with the rest for about thirty seconds. Add about 150 ml (3/4 cup) of milk and some candy sugar (optional). Boil everything together for another minute. Your stimulating and rejuvenating tea is ready. This drink is a very effective substitute to replace coffee.

*Long pepper is called *Piper longum* in Latin and *pippali* in Hindi. If you do not get it abroad, replace it with normal black pepper.

Breakfast: You need two tablespoons of black chickpeas, also called black gram (*kala chana* in Hindi), soaked in water for 24 hours prior to consumption. These can be eaten as such but chew them well. Alternatively, fry these with a teaspoon of sesame oil and some cumin. You can drink another cup of Rejuvenating tea with this. You can also add some milk in the tea.

Lunch: Make mixed vegetable Recipe Number 1. Eat this with plain rice* or steamed potatoes. Take a fruit for dessert but not banana.

Dinner: Make mixed vegetable recipe Number 2 and eat it with two pieces of bread or two *chapatis***. You can also eat a preparation of wheat, millet or

---

* It is a preparation of rice without salt or fat. The rice is cooked in water and some spices. Recipe is given on the following pages.
* *The best is if you can make chapatis or bread with barley flour. You can mix 2/3 of barley with 1/3 of wheat flower. Barley has quality of decreasing bulk. Recipe is given on the following pages.

another grain. Do not eat maize bread, as it is highly bulk promoting. For dessert, eat either a fruit (not banana) or a piece of chocolate (15 gm only) or a sweet preparation of sesames seeds. But remember to eat only a small piece.

Day 2

Morning drink: As described above.

Breakfast: Take 100 gm paneer or cottage cheese with fresh tomatoes, carrots or apple. Alternatively, take one glass (200ml) of full-cream milk with one sweet apple or a carrot. If you do not like milk products, take a preparation of *sattu* (explanation and recipe given later). Alternatively, you can prepare a vegetable and fruit juice or a fruit salad. There should be no salt or sugar in this breakfast.

Lunch: Mung bean sprouts mixed salad along with either two pieces of bread or chapatis. Take figs or papaya or mango for dessert.

Dinner: Take Carrot soup or massor dal soup along with bread or chapatis. Take dates for dessert.

Day 3

Morning drink: Take the morning rejuvenating tea or other warm drinks you are used to. Preserved juices should not be taken. A warm drink is recommended.

Breakfast: Take 200 gm (a cup) of plane full-cream yoghurt with two teaspoons of honey in it. You can take it without honey if you wish to cut a fruit like apple or mango in your yoghurt. If you are averse to dairy products, take sattu or kala chana breakfast.

Lunch: Eat plain basmati rice along with a preparation of mixed vegetable Number 3. Take a fruit for dessert (not banana).

Dinner: Take a preparation of mixed vegetables 4 or 5 along with a preparation of dalia with sesame seeds. Take some raisins for dessert. You can also take dried raisins.

Day 4

Morning drink: Take the morning drink as usual.

Breakfast: Take papaya and banana for breakfast. Take 2 small bananas or one big banana and about 500 gm (1 Pound) of papaya.

Lunch: Take curd-rice for lunch and slices of cucumber along side as a salad. But there should be no oily or fatty sauce on the cucumber. Eat some dates for dessert.

Dinner: Make a preparation of semolina with mixed vegetables as described in the recipes. You may prepare the spring onion salad or other salads without oil and with only lemon juice. Alternatively, you can take Mung dal or pumpkin soup instead of a salad. Take a fruit for dessert (not banana).

Day 5

This is a special day on which you will not take any salt and grains like wheat, millet, rice, etc.

Morning drink: Take your morning drink as usual.

Breakfast: Grate finely 2 to 3 medium sized carrots. Cook them by adding 2 tablespoons of water. Cook with the lid on at very low fire for 15 minutes and stir from time to time. Add 2 cardamoms into it after removing them from pods. Add about 150 ml (3/4 cup) of milk into the carrots. Cook for 2-3 minutes more. In case you do not want milk, replace it with ½ teaspoon of ghee (clarified butter) or butter in the end.

Lunch: Eat a preparation of green peas and paneer (recipe to make paneer is given later in the chapter). Cook about 100 gm of green peas in very little water along with some cumin, fresh ginger, a pinch of pepper and some dill seeds. Cook them covered until the peas are soft. Separately, smear a non-stick pan with ghee and roast the pieces of paneer made from half litre milk. Add the green peas preparation into it and you have a nice looking food plate ready.

Eat an apple or another sweet fruit for dessert.

Dinner: Make vegetable Number 6. Eat this with either boiled potatoes or vapour the potatoes in a non-stick pan with lid after smearing it with little ghee.

Eat ten peeled almonds with a little honey or some dates or a fruit for dessert.

Day 6

Morning drink: Take your morning drink as usual.

Breakfast: Take fruits for breakfast.

Lunch: Take vegetable Number 7 along with germinated wheat bread. Eat a piece of papaya or some other fruit for dessert.

Dinner: Take a mixed vegetable soup with dalia preparation or two slices of bread. Eat some raisins or dates or figs for dessert.

Day 7

Morning drink: Take your morning drink as usual.

Breakfast: Make the carrots as described for Day 5. But do not add milk in them. Add a tablespoon of chopped almonds. You may add ½ teaspoon of sugar if you wish. Normally, carrots are sweet and one does not need sugar in this preparation. Add a pinch of saffron into the preparation.

Lunch: Make green rice preparation and eat this with spring onion salad or another similar mixed salad prepared without or with very little olive oil. Alternatively, you can eat this with banana or cucumber rayata (a yoghurt preparation). Eat figs or other fruits for dessert.

Dinner: Make vegetable Number 8 along with germinated wheat bread or some grain preparation. Take a fruit for dessert.

The Diet Recipes*

Breakfast

Germinated chickpea breakfast

This breakfast gives you strength and not bulk. In fact, dark chickpeas, which are slightly smaller in size than the normal chickpeas but similar in shape and are brown in colour are highly strength promoting. They are used as diet for horses. In France and perhaps also in other European countries, they can be bought at the shops where they sell horse food.

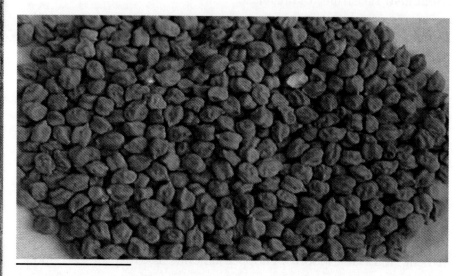

* I have given a list of bulk promoting and bulk reducing food products in the Appendix. Besides following the recipes given for the diet plan, pay attention to the food products you take thereafter in order to maintain the right weight.

They are also available in Indian or oriental shops.

Ingredients for one person:

Black gram or black chickpeas 3 to 4 tablespoons

Soak chickpeas in water for 24 hours after washing them a few times. They become soft and edible. Wash them with water and eat them as such. Chew them properly. If you find them hard, smear the non stick pan with little ghee, add some cumin and a little salt and cook them for 10 minutes with the lid on.

Breakfast with sattu

Sattu is made from roasted black chickpeas or roasted barley. It is very popular in North India. It is very tasteful and invigorating. Roasted grains are bulk reducing. Powder the roasted black chickpeas or barley and then mix this powder with hot or cold water. This powder is called sattu. Add 2-3 tablespoons of sattu and pour hot or cold water on it. Whip a little to mix well. Sweeten it with candy sugar to taste. It becomes like a thick soup.

In India, sattu can be bought ready made. It is possible to get roasted black chickpeas on Indian shops abroad. You can grind them yourself to make sattu.

Soups

Mung dal soup

Ingredients for 2 to 3 portions:

Mung dal*	100gm (½ cup)
Carrot	2 medium sized
Fresh spinach	100 gm (¼ lb.)
Water	500 ml (2 ½ cup)

* Mung dal is mung beans split, and without husk. It is available in the shops as mung dal. It is yellow in colour.

Fresh lemon juice	1 tablespoon
Salt	¼ teaspoon or to taste
Pepper	a pinch
Coriander	¼ teaspoon
Cumin	¼ teaspoon
Fennel	¼ teaspoon
Turmeric	1 teaspoon
Ghee	1 teaspoon
Chopped basil	1 tablespoon

Add in a pot chopped spinach and carrots, cleaned and washed mung dal, spices and about 300 ml (1 ½ cup) water. Cook for about 20 minutes to half an hour, on low heat, half covered and stir from time to time. Make sure that the dal is well cooked as the time of cooking may vary according to the quality of the water. In the end, add some more water to make it fluid and bring it to boil. The quantity of the water you add depends upon the consistency of the soup you would like to have. Add salt and lemon juice. You may decide to blend it with a hand blender or serve it as such. Add ghee before serving. Add chopped basil on the top before serving.

Carrot soup

Ingredients for 2 or 3 portions:

Carrots	1/2 Kg (1 lb.)
Potato	1 medium sized
Water	400 ml (2 cups)
Chopped green herbs	4 tablespoons
Coriander	¼ teaspoon
Cumin	¼ teaspoon
Fennel	¼ teaspoon
Salt	¼ teaspoon
Turmeric	½ teaspoon
Ghee or butter	1 teaspoon
Fresh green herbs	1 tablespoon (finely chopped)

Wash, peel and chop the carrots and the potato. Put them in a pot along with water. Bring them to boil and add fresh herbs, spices and salt. Cook them covered on a slow fire until the vegetables are soft. Blend the cooked contents with the hand mixer and add ghee or butter before serving

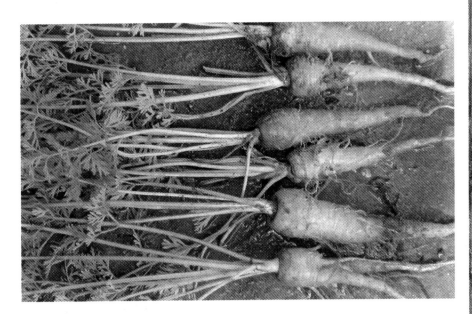

Mixed vegetable soup

Mixed vegetable soup may be prepared with different vegetables of your choice like green peas, carrots, broccoli, spinach, tomatoes, cabbage and so on. You may add a little of each vegetable.

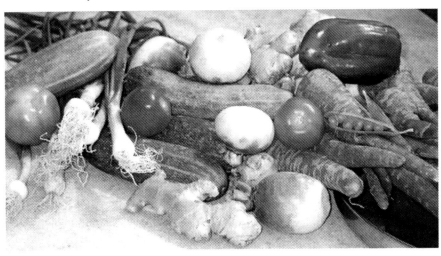

Ingredients for 2 to 3 portions:

Carrot	1 medium sized
Broccoli	100 gm (¼ lb.)
Potato	1 medium sized
Green peas	3 tablespoons
Tomatoes	2 medium sized
Water	300 ml (1 ½ cup)
Salt	¼ teaspoon
Pepper	a pinch
Nutmeg	¼ of a nut (freshly grated)
Cumin	½ teaspoon
Coriander	¼ teaspoon
Fennel	¼ teaspoon
Fresh herbs chopped	1 tablespoon
Ghee or butter	1 teaspoon

Cut all the vegetable into fine pieces and put them all accept tomatoes in a pot and cook them for about 15 minutes on low heat after it comes to boil. Keep the pot covered. Add tomatoes, salt and the spices accept nutmeg and cook for another 10-15 minutes on reduced heat and with the lid on. Add the nutmeg in the end. Add ghee or butter before serving and decorate it with fresh herbs.

Red lentil (masoor dal) soup

Ingredients for 3 to 4 portions:

Red lentils	150 gm (¾ cup)
Carrots	4 medium sized
Tomatoes	5 medium sized
Onions	2 medium sized
Garlic	4 to 6 cloves
Water	1 Litre (5 cups)
Coriander	¼ teaspoon
Cumin	¼ teaspoon
Fennel	¼ teaspoon

Salt	1/3 to ½ teaspoon
Turmeric	1 teaspoon
Butter or ghee	2 teaspoon

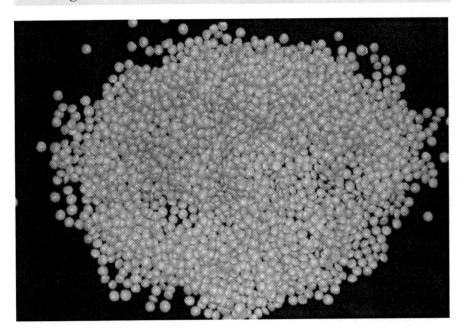

Wash and soak the lentils for about 10 minutes in water. Take a big pot of two litres so that it is half full when you add water. Bring the water to boil and add lentils after draining out the water in which they were soaking. Add turmeric and bring it to boil. Go on adding carrots cut into small pieces and when everything is boiling, reduce the heat and let it cook slowly for 15 minutes. Then add to it tomatoes cut into small pieces and onions in lamellae. Add also the rest of the spices and salt except garlic. Let everything cook for another 15 minutes on low heat after it comes to boil. Depending on the quality of water, you may have to cook a little longer or add a little more water. Add garlic when the soup is ready and turn off the heat. Add butter or ghee in the end before serving.

Pumpkin soup

Ingredients for 2 to 3 portions:	
Pumpkin	400 gm (1lb.)

Water	200 ml (1 cup)
Salt	¼ teaspoon
Cumin	½ teaspoon
Small cardamom	4
Pepper	6-7 seeds
Dill seeds	¼ teaspoon
Milk	100 ml (½ cup)

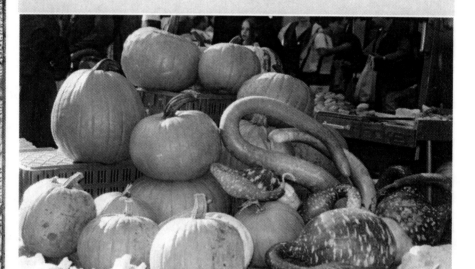

Peel and cut the pumpkin into small pieces and cook it in water with the lid on and on low heat until it is completely soft. Remove the pods of the cardamom and powder all the four spices in a mortar. Add the spices and the salt into the pot and cook for another 2 minutes. Add milk, stir everything together and bring it to boil. Let it cool a little and mix it with a hand mixer. Add a little butter in each portion before serving.

Vegetable preparations

Some general instructions for cooking vegetables

The best way to do low fat cooking is in a non-stick pan with a lid. The cooking should be done at low heat with the lid on. Salt should be added in the end so that the vegetables do not absorb the salt and your salt intake is low.

Vegetable Number 1

Mixed vegetables with raisins

This is a recipe without salt. Generally people are extremely unhappy when they are supposed to eat food without salt due to an ailment or regimen. Try this recipe and you will realise that sometimes vegetables without salt can taste better than with salt.

Ingredients for 2 to 3 portions:

Carrots	3 medium-sized
Green peas	4 tablespoons
Beans	100 gm (¼ lb.)
Cauliflower	100 gm (¼ lb.)
Paprika	1 medium-sized
Ginger (chopped)	3 tablespoons
Cumin	½ teaspoon
Fennel	½ teaspoon
Cardamom	4
Clove	4
Ghee or cooking oil	2 teaspoons
Raisins	1 tablespoon

Cut the vegetables into small pieces and keep each of them separately. Paprika should be cut into long pieces. Grind all the four spices together after removing pods from the cardamom. Heat the oil in a pot and add beans into it. Stir a little and then put the lid on and reduce the heat. Beans take longer to cook than the rest of the vegetables and that is why they need prior cooking. After about 10 minutes, add carrots, peas, cauliflower and ginger into it. Stir everything together and cook for another 10 minutes with the lid on. Keep stirring from time to time. The vegetables cook with their own vapours when cooked with the lid on and on low heat. Add the powdered spices and raisins and stir everything together. Cook for another two minutes and it is ready.

Vegetable Number 2

Mixed vegetables with spices

This is a very simple recipe that is made with a combination of uncrushed spices

Ingredients for 2 to 3 portions:

Green cabbage	200 gm (½ lb.) (Finely chopped)
Green peas	100 gm (¼ lb)
Carrots	2 medium-sized (chopped thin and round)
Paprika	1 (chopped fine and long)
Sesames or olive oil	2 teaspoons
Salt	¼ teaspoon or to taste
Green chilli	¼ to ½ (optional)
Fresh lemon juice	1 teaspoon (optional)
Spice mixture*	1 teaspoon

*The spice mixture has the following ingredients:

Coriander, fennel, fenugreek, mustard seeds, cumin, and kalonji, mixed in equal quantities.

Heat the oil in a pan or a wok. When it is hot enough, add the spice mixture. After a few seconds, add salt and chilli and then add vegetables. Go on stirring so that the spices can mix well with the vegetables. Cook uncovered for first five minutes while stirring from time to time. Cook covered on a very low heat for another five minutes. Remove the lid and stir on medium heat to make the vegetable crisp. Add lemon juice in the end and stir. However, the addition of lemon juice is optional. Some of you may not like it sour and can leave out lemon juice.

Suggestions: You may replace cabbage with cauliflower or broccoli.

Vegetable Number 3

Carrots and green peas

Carrots are a very good food from the Ayurvedic point of view as they create equilibrium of the three energies of the body.

Ingredients for 2 portions:

Carrots	4 medium-sized
Young green peas	100 to 150 gm (½ to ¾ Cup)
Onion	1 medium-sized
Ginger	1 tablespoon
Turmeric	¼ teaspoon
Salt	a pinch
Cumin	½ teaspoon
Fennel	¼ teaspoon
Coriander	¼ teaspoon
Ghee or olive oil	1 teaspoon

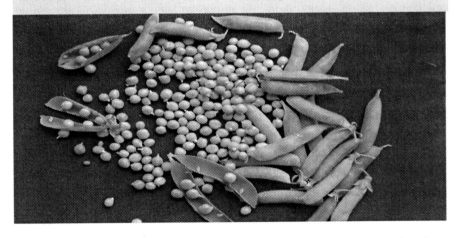

Cut ginger and onions into small pieces and fry them in ghee or oil. When the onions are sauté, add all the spices and the salt and stir everything together. Add carrots cut into small pieces and young green peas. Stir to mix everything together. Reduce the heat and cook the vegetables with a lid on the pot. The cooking time is about 15 minutes. Keep stirring from time to time.

Vegetable number 4
Pumpkin

Ingredients for 2 portions:

Pumpkin	about ½ Kg (1 Pound)
Sesames or olive oil	1 teaspoon
Spice Mixture*	½ teaspoon
Salt	¼ teaspoon
Turmeric	½ teaspoon
Mango powder or lemon juice	½ teaspoon

* The spice mixture has the following ingredients:

Coriander, fennel, fenugreek, mustard seeds, cumin, and kalonji, mixed in equal quantities.

Peel, clean (get rid of the seeds etc.) and cut the pumpkin into small pieces. Heat oil in a wok or a pot and add the spices and salt (except mango powder or lemon juice). Add the pumpkin pieces and mix everything together. Put the lid on and reduce the heat. Cook for about 15 minutes. Stir once or twice in between. Normally pumpkin has plenty of water. Cook until the pumpkin pieces are completely soft. Remove the lid and add mango powder or lemon juice. Stir and cook for another 5 minutes. This preparation should not be very watery. Cook a little longer while stirring so that the water evaporates.

This recipe is sweet and sour tasting. In case your pumpkin is raw and it does not taste sweet, you may add a little raw sugar into it.

Vegetable Number 5

String beans with ginger

There is no fat at all in this preparation.

Ingredients for 2 to 3 portions:

String beans	200gm (½ lb.)
Water	100 ml (½ cup)
Tomatoes	2 medium-sized
Salt	¼ teaspoon
Ginger (small pieces)	1 tablespoon
Cumin	½ teaspoon
Cardamom	4

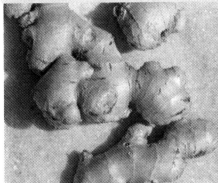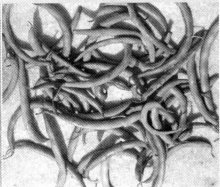

Put the water into a pot and bring it to boil. Cut the beans into small pieces and put them in boiling water. Cook for 15-20 minutes on low heat with the lid on. Stir from time to time and add a little more water if needed. Add tomatoes, ginger and spices and cook for another 10 minutes. Cardamoms should be added after taking them out from the pods and crushing a little

Vegetable Number 6

Spinach with tomatoes

Ingredients for 2 to 3 portions:

Spinach	200 gm
Tomatoes	2 medium sized
Onion	1 medium sized
Oil or ghee	1 ½ teaspoon
Clove	4
Cardamom	3
Coriander	¼ teaspoon
Fennel	¼ teaspoon
Turmeric	½ teaspoon
Cumin	½ teaspoon
Ginger (chopped)	1 teaspoon
Garlic	two cloves
Chooped coriander* (herb)	1 teaspoon

*If you do not have coriander, replace it with parsley.

Either make spinach purée after cooking spinach in water for about 15 minutes and mixing it with hand mixer or use as such. Make a sauce by first frying onions and when they are sauté, add the spices, stir for a minute and add finely chopped tomatoes. Cook everything while stirring until the tomatoes are well cooked. Add the cooked spinach into it cook everything together for about 10 minutes while stirring. Add crushed ginger, garlic and herbs in the end.

Vegetable Number 7

Turnips with green peas

Turnip is another vegetable that brings equilibrium in the body.

Ingredients for 2 to 3 portions:

Turnips	3-4 medium sized
Green peas	100 gm (½ cup)
Onion	1 medium-sized
Olive or sesames	1 teaspoon
Salt	a pinch
Clove	4
Cardamom	3
Coriander	¼ teaspoon
Fennel	¼ teaspoon
Turmeric	½ teaspoon
Cumin	½ teaspoon

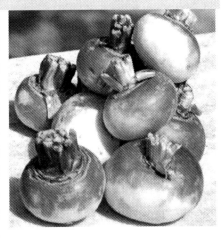

Cut the onion into small pieces. Peel and cut the turnips also into small pieces. Heat the ghee and add onions into it. When onions are sauté, add the spices and salt and stir. Add turnips now and mix everything well. Reduce the heat, put the lid on and let them cook on low heat for 10 minutes. Stir from time to time to make sure that the preparation does not stick to the bottom. Add pre-cooked green peas and stir them with the rest. Cook for another 5 minutes.

Vegetable Number 8

Courgette or zucchini

Here is a simple preparation of courgette (as well as of *tori* and lauki found in India) with tomatoes.

Ingredients for 2 to 3 portions:

Courgette or other similar vegetables	½ Kilo (1 lb)
Ginger (small pieces)	1 tablespoon
Tomatoes	4 medium-sized
Water	200 ml (1 cup)
Salt	¼ teaspoon
Spice Mixture*	½ teaspoon
Chopped green herbs	1 teaspoon
Ghee or butter	1 teaspoon

* Coriander, fennel, fenugreek, mustard seeds, cumin, and kalonji, mixed in equal quantities.

This is a kind of recipe you can make when you are short of time and are unable to pay full attention at each step of the preparation. Cut all the vegetables into small pieces and put everything in a pot excluding ghee. Put water in the pot first, then courgette. Sprinkle the pieces of ginger on the top of courgette, then all the spices including salt. Cover the spices with the pieces of tomatoes and put the lid on. Let everything cook on a low heat for about 20 minutes with the lid on. Stir once after about 15 minutes. Add ghee or butter in the end.

Some other preparations

Semolina with vegetables (uppama)

Ingredients for 2 to 3 portions:

Semolina	100 gm (½ cup)
Chopped ginger	1 tablespoon
Paprika	2 medium sized
Carrots	2 medium sized
Green peas (tender)	3 tablespoons
Tomatoes	2 medium sized
Fresh ginger (chopped)	1 tablespoon
Green herbs (chopped)	1 tablespoon
Salt	½ to ¾ teaspoon
Cumin	1 teaspoon
Mustard seeds	½ teaspoon
Sesames or olive oil	1 ½ teaspoon

Cut paprika and tomatoes into small pieces but keep them separately. Grate the carrots. Heat the oil in a pot and add cumin and mustard seeds. Reduce the heat and add salt and rest of the spices including ginger. Fry for 20 seconds and add paprika, carrots and peas and stir-fry. After about 5 minutes, add tomatoes and stir-fry another 5 minutes. Add semolina and stir everything together for about a minute. Add gradually thrice the quantity of water than semolina. Keep stirring and bring it to boil. Reduce the heat and stir from time to time. Semolina soaks water very quickly and the dish is ready after about 30 seconds of adding water.

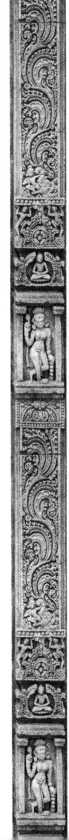

Plain rice

Ingredients for 2 portions:

Basmati rice	½ cup or whatever measure you use (about 100 gm)*
Water	1 cup (or twice the quantity of the rice with the measure you have used)
Cardamom	2
Clove	3

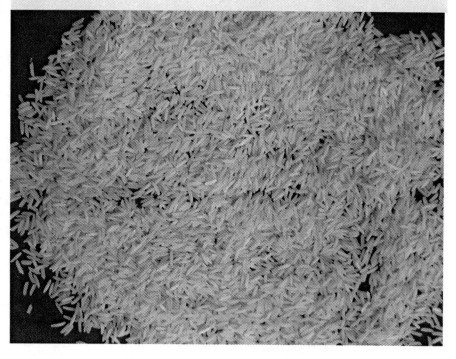

You always need double the amount of water to cook rice. You may measure your rice with any glass or cup and simply take double the quantity of water. Wash the rice properly and then soak it in water from 10 to 15 minutes. For plain rice preparation, put the water in a pot with a thick

---

* Rice is not taken by weight but by measure (volume). If you wish to cook 200 gm of rice (half pound), which is generally enough for three persons, measure it with a glass or any other container and measure the quantity of the water with the same container. You always require twice the volume of water to cook rice.

bottom. Add cardamom after removing the pods and cloves. Cover the water, bring it to boil and then add the soaked rice in it after draining out completely the water they were soaked in. Do it with a strainer. When all the rice is in boiling water, reduce to very low heat and cover it. Let the rice cook very slowly. After about 8 minutes (or a little more, depending upon the quality and age of rice and quality of water), you will smell the fine perfume of Basmati. Put off the heat and let the pot remain as such. Put a little weight or a napkin to cover the lid so that the vapours do not escape. Let it lie for about five minutes like this before serving. Rice should always be cooked a little before they are served.

Quantity of rice: For the diet meals, you are suggested to take 50 gm (¼ cup) of rice per person.

Green rice

Ingredients for 2 portions:

Basmati rice	½ cup (about 100 gm)
Water	1 cup (200 ml)
Various green, leafy vegetables (Finely chopped)	200 gm (½ pound)
Onion	1 medium sized
Cumin	1 teaspoon
Cardamom	4
Salt	¼ teaspoon or to taste.
Olive or sesames oil	1 teaspoon

Wash and soak the rice for at least 10 minutes. Fry the onions in oil briefly and then add cumin, cardamom and salt. Stir everything together and go on adding green vegetables while stirring. Cook the vegetables on low fire with the lid on the pot for about five minutes. Uncover and stir again in order to get rid of excessive water if any. Add washed and soaked rice into the vegetables after draining out the water. Stir gently and add boiling water. Put the lid on and cook on a low fire. After about 8 or 9 minutes, when you have the fragrance of the basmati rice, turn off the heat and leave the preparation as such for another 5 minutes. Put a napkin on the pot so that it maintains its heat. This preparation looks green due to the predominant colour of the green vegetables.

Curd-rice

According to Ayurveda, yoghurt is nectar when eaten in the morning, good at noon and poison at night. Thus, this preparation should be exclusively eaten for breakfast or lunch.

Ingredients for 2 to 3 portions:

Rice	100 gm (½ cup)
Yoghurt	400 gm (2 cups)
Sesame or olive oil	2 teaspoons
Cumin	1 teaspoon
Mustard seeds	1 teaspoon
Salt	½ teaspoon or according to taste
Fresh coriander leaves (chopped)	1 tablespoon
Ajwain	½ teaspoon
Grated coconut	2 tablespoon
Pomegranate fruit	1 (optional)

Wash and soak the rice and cook it in water as described for the plain rice. Put it on the side and let it cool. Heat oil in a pot and when it is very hot, add cumin and mustard seeds in it, reduce the heat and fry for about 20 seconds. Put off the heat and add immediately grated coconut, salt, ajwain and coriander leaves, and stir. Mix all this with the rice. Separately, whip the yoghurt and prepare pomegranate seeds. Add these two ingredients to the rice. Make sure that the rice is at room temperature.

Dalia* with sesame seeds

Ingredients for two portions:

Dalia	100 gm (½ cup)
Water	300 ml (1 ½ cup)

**Dalia is crushed wheat. It is available in Indian grocery shops abroad. In Turkish and other oriental shops it is called Bulgar.

Salt	a pinch
Cumin	½ teaspoon
Ghee	1 teaspoon
Sesame seeds	1 teaspoon

Heat the oil in a pot and add cumin seeds first and then a few seconds later add dalia. Roast dalia by stirring it for a minute or two on medium heat. Add water and salt and reduce the fire. Let it cook for about 10 minutes on low heat. Add sesame seeds, stir a little and cover the preparation again. Cook until the grains are soft. Like rice, consider measuring dalia rather than weighing it and take three times the water with the same measure. It may be possible that the dalia or the bulgar you have has bigger grains or is of another variety. Keep in mind that the grain should be soft. Uncooked grains disturb vata energy of the body.

Rayatas

Rayatas are principally made of yoghurt (called curd in India) along with some vegetables or fruits and spices for flavouring. Remember that yoghurt should not be eaten at night and thus, the rayatas should not be taken for dinner.

Banana rayata

Ingredients for 2 portions:

Yoghurt	200 gm (1 cup)
Bananas	2 medium-sized
Salt	a pinch
Pepper	a pinch
Cumin	½ teaspoon

Whip the yoghurt a little after adding salt and pepper. Cut bananas into roundels and put into the yoghurt. Stir with a spoon and mix well. Put cumin on a heated pan, stir a little with a wooden spoon for about 20 seconds or until it is slightly roasted. Put the roasted cumin in a mortar and crush to powder. Add this to the rayata and mix.

Cucumber rayata

In this rayata, replace the banana with small pieces of cucumber. Take cucumber and yoghurt in equal parts. Instead of cumin, add some finely chopped fresh mint leaves or crushed dried mint.

Making paneer from milk

Paneer can be compared to fresh cheese. Solids of the milk are separated by adding some sour substance in the boiling milk. Take a litre of full cream fresh milk, put it in a pot and heat it. Wait until it comes to a boil. At this stage, add immediately a tablespoon of lemon juice. The solids of the milk will begin to float in the semi-transparent liquid. In case you do not see the semi-transparent liquid separate from the solids of the milk, it means you require a little more lemon juice. Add a little more lemon juice and wait and see. Do not add immediately the second entire soupspoon full of lemon juice. When you see the solids of the milk in lumps in the watery substance, your paneer is ready.

Normally one tablespoon full of lemon juice is enough to make paneer from 1 litre (5 cups) of fresh milk but due to the pasteurisation and homogenisation of the milk in many places in the world, you may require a little more lemon juice than that.

For the above described diet recommendations, you need to separate the solids from the liquid. For that, pass the contents through a thin muslin cloth and hang it to drain out the rest of the water. For making cubes, put the whole thing (paneer inside the cloth) on a flat surface like a wooden board and put on it a flat-bottomed pot full of water or any other weight you can think of. This is done to squeeze out the rest of the fluid and obtain a solid piece, which holds together and can be cut into small cubes.

A litre of good full cream milk gives rise to between 200 to 250 gm of paneer.

Salads

Spring Onion Salad

Ingredients for 2 to 3 portions:

Spring onions	200 gm (½ lb)
Paprika	1 medium-sized
Tomato	1 medium sized
Apple	1
Coriander leaves or	2 tablespoons
Other herbs chopped	
Rock salt	1/4 teaspoon
Pepper	1 pinch
Lemon juice	1 ½ tablespoon

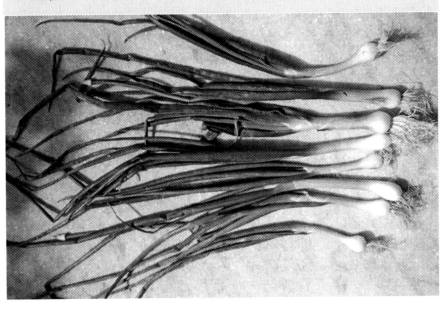

Cut the spring onions very fine and do not use the lower green part, as it too fibrous for being eaten raw. However, you may keep it for soup. Cut tomatoes, apple and paprika into very fine pieces. Mix everything including green herbs. Add salt and pepper into lemon juice and mix. This should be added to the salad just before serving.

Breads

Germinated wheat bread

Ingredients for 3 or 4 flat breads like the pancakes:

Wheat grains	250 gm
Salt (Optional)	1/4 teaspoon
Ajwain	½ teaspoon
Kalonji	1/4 teaspoon
Ghee or cooking oil	2 teaspoons

Germinate the wheat by soaking it in water for 24 hours. The grains should be just at the beginning of germination. Wash and crush the germinated wheat in a wet grinder. Add a few tablespoons of water if it is too dry for grinding. Take out the crushed wheat and add salt and spices into it.

Mix the spices in the crushed grains. Heat a non-stick pan smeared with a little ghee. When it is very hot, put 2 to 3 tablespoons of the dough (it is something between dough and batter in consistency) on it and spread it with a wooden flat spoon. After about half a minute, reduce the heat and let the bread cook slowly. Put the wooden spoon under the sides of the bread to make sure it is not sticking. After about a minute, turn the bread over and add a little more ghee on the pan. Let it cook on medium fire until both sides of the bread are light brown. Normally, if you are patient, you will have to turn the bread over only one time. The important factor in making this bread is that the dough should be spread properly on the pan to make thin bread. Thick bread takes quite long to cook and sometimes remains uncooked in the middle.

Comments: You can also make the bread without any spices. With the sweet taste of the germinated wheat, it is delicious.

Chapati

Chapati is the simplest form of flat bread with just whole-wheat flour and water, it is baked on a pan without any fat. It is suggested to make chapatis with barley flour mixed 50% with wheat flour as barley is bulk decreasing. Chapati is always made fresh and eaten hot. The dough is made by adding water little by little into the flour and kneading for some time. After kneading, the dough becomes elastic and does not remain sticky. The dough should be kept for about 15 minutes before making chapatis.

Take nearly one tablespoon of dough between your palms and make a ball from it. Flatten it first by pressing it between your palms and then with a rolling pin. Use some flour for preventing it from sticking on the surface while rolling. Roll it as thin as possible. Pick it up very carefully and put it on a pre-heated pan. Turn it over after a few seconds. Turn it over once again after about 20-30 seconds and press the surface gently with a cotton napkin. By doing so, chapati will puff up. It is now ready.

Comments: You can add some ajwain seeds in chapati dough especially during winter months.

Barley Roti

Roti is like chapatti and it has the same recipe as described above for the chapatti but it is thicker than chapatti and therefore does not puff up so well. As has been said earlier, barley is bulk reducing and therefore I recommend highly to use barley roti to replace bread or other wheat preparations. Use the above-described recipe for chapatti.

Alternatively, you can also make a thick batter of barley flour, add cumin seeds, salt and finely chopped onions and some herbs and make in a similar manner as described for the germinated wheat bread.

3

Soft Methods for Losing Weight

Discipline and patience are the two key words for losing weight with soft or gentle methods. This is the way to lose weight very gradually over a long period of time by fundamentally changing your lifestyle and food habits. These methods are recommended more to those persons who are moderately overweight and do not like to go through the efforts of making a special diet to get rid of the weight.

Age is an important factor. If you are already a little overweight during your childhood and youth, the danger is to get excessively overweight around the age of 50 or let us call it the middle age. The over weight at that age accompanies also various ailments and disorders. Therefore, I recommend using the soft methods of losing weight to this category of persons.

Through discipline, you should avoid all the weight-enhancing factors given in Chapter 1 of this Section. Besides that, I recommend the following four major methods in a comprehensive manner in order to lose weight gradually and attain health and vitality:

1.   Changing your lifestyle
2.   Changing your food habits
3.   Alternating your menus daily
4.   Disciplined sleeping hours

Changing your lifestyle

Lead a disciplined lifestyle which is well organised and not haphazard. I give you the following suggestions:

☐ Make an effort to get up at a more or less fixed time. What I mean to say is if you are used to getting up at 7 in the morning, try not to get up later than 8 also on days you have no engagements or work schedule. Do not drastically alter body's sleeping rhythm.

☐ Make it a habit to drink a glass of hot water immediately after getting up.

☐ After drinking hot water, take a walk or do yoga at least for 10 minutes, preferably for 15 minutes.

☐ Make sure you evacuate properly. In case you evacuate only partially or suffer from mild constipation, drink more hot water in the morning followed by hot tea or coffee or any other hot drink you are used to. If still it does not work, make sure to eat a vegetable soup for dinner and take a mild purgative if needed.

☐ Never ever sit down after your meals. If you are pressed for time after lunch, move around at least for five minutes. It is even more important to walk and be active after dinner.

☐ Have your dinner three hours before going to bed. Try to be disciplined about meal times and never ever eat between meals. More details of nutrition and food culture are given in Section III, Chapter 2.

☐ Make a mental effort to get rid of inertia and lethargy. Do not postpone doing things and try to establish an order around you. Use your will power against leading a sedentary lifestyle.

Changing your food habits

Right weight is the sign of health and overweight amounts to putting extra stress on your body organs and thus cutting short your lifespan (see the citation from Charaka in the beginning of the book). When I use the word 'overweight', I do not really mean obese. Even two to three kilos of overweight is harmful.

For reducing weight gradually over a long period of time is actually based on the principle of changing your lifestyle and food habits and integrating the suggested ways in your life forever. However, it does not mean that you should lead an austere life. You can go to wild parties or big dinners or eat rich and good meals from time to time. But you have to live in such a planned way that you are prepared to give an antidote to the excesses immediately after, for regaining harmony and balance.

I have given several menus in the second chapter and you may follow that pattern and make sure that your meals are enriched with various elements and rasas (tastes) and should include a variety of things. They should be tasty and the use of spices and herbs is very essential to enrich them. For more detail of the variety of delicious recipes and spice mixtures, refer to my book, *Ayurvedic Food Culture and Recipes*.

You can make the recipes given in my food book or your own recipes by taking care of the following points:

- ☐ Cook the vegetable recipes in non-stick pan with ½ to 1/3 of the fat you normally use.

- ☐ Make your meals with a variety of vegetables and use very little ghee or oil to cook them. Use spices like cardamom, cumin, pepper, fennel, coriander seeds, curcuma (turmeric) fenugreek, nutmeg, mace, ginger and garlic, Cook the vegetables covered in a non-stick pan or other similar pan with the lid on. Cook always on low heat and let them simmer and cook in their own water.

- ☐ Accompanying the vegetables should be either cheese or something made of grains like pasta, bread or chapati or rice. The grains and cheese should not be together. Grain preparations should be eaten once a day and the other meal should be taken with cheese or potatoes.

- ☐ Meat eaters should avoid heavy and fatty meats and should stick to chicken soup, fish and seafood.

Weekly partial fast: Once a week, on the same day every week, observe a partial fast day. This is not a fast in the sense of staying hungry it is simply to eat different food in a controlled manner. The suggested diet for this special day is given in the box below.

Food for Partial fast day

You can eat fruits, vegetables, nuts, yoghurt, milk and cheese. No preparations made of grains (e.g. rice, barley, wheat, maize, lentils, beans and so on) and no salt should be taken on this day. Do not eat onions, garlic and other strong spices like chillies, etc. Pepper can be taken. Meat and eggs and anything else that is not vegetarian should not be eaten.

For breakfast you can have any of these things: cheese, nuts, fruits, yoghurt and milk. Your choice of cheese is restricted to the unsalted fresh cheese as most processed cheeses have salt in them.

If you have to work physically hard or walk a lot, you can have fruits like bananas and papaya or eat some nuts or cheese for lunch as well. Otherwise eat an early dinner.

For the evening meal, you may prepare a plate of fresh vegetables by using a few herbs and spices like cumin, thyme, fennel seeds, ginger and cardamom. You can eat these with a potato preparation but always remember not to add salt in anything.

Partial fasting helps to revitalise the digestive system. By eating less and eating things that have high water contents and not taking any salt, the body purifies it self and releases extra water. Balance of water in the body is very crucial for losing weight.

Food consumption and S-Factor: Here are some more instructions regarding your food intake that will help you balance weight through discipline.

☐   Discipline yourself never to overeat. Always 2/3 stomach full. If you are used to eating full stomach, it will need an initial effort to get used to the healthy way of keeping the stomach partially empty for the process of digestion.

☐   Never ever eat between meals⁻ not even 'something little'. Have an early, complete and satisfying meal.

☐   Use of spices described above and fresh herbs to enrich your meals with S-Factor (see Chapter 1, number 7 of this section). These provide you the subtle energy (prana) and with a sense of satisfaction. Many times, we eat more because we are not satisfied with the taste. We feel full but not fulfilled. In that process, we feel like eating more even after a complete meal. Spices provide you rasayanas or vitality-enhancing S-factor and give satisfaction without enhanced fat and sweet.

Alternating your menu daily

Alternate your menu from one day to the other in terms of nutrition. This is a trick of nature that the same things may make you put on weight if eaten regularly whereas if you alter your diet from one day to the other; no matter if it is with the same amount of calories, the bulk promoting effect is reduced. For example, one day if you are eating low fat diet with rice, vegetables, potatoes and fruits, the next day, your diet should be dominant in dairy products. Again next day, alter your diet with barley or millet bread and soup with a little olive oil or ghee in it. The effect on weight does not work exclusively with calories. The fat eaten between these two different menus does not enhance your weight. However, if three days in a row you take dairy products and then three days the vegetables and bread menu, you will put on more weight as compared to altering nutrition everyday.

Disciplined sleeping hours

Sleep contributes to overweight. You should be very disciplined and should never sleep late or during the day. Change in food habits can solve this problem. If you eat less fatty and heavy food, you tend to sleep less. Thus, when you follow the above-described instructions about diet, you will automatically sleep less. Similarly, use of spices like garlic, ginger, pepper and cumin reduce sleep requirement.

If you have a habit of sleeping a lot, use your will power to adopt a more active way of life. Night is meant for sleeping and our body is timed in such a way that during night, its energy channels partially close. After 6-7 hours of good and sound sleep, one feels refreshed. If one sleeps more than that, it makes an individual tired and lazy. In the present context of shaping yourself, you should not forget that sleeping more than body's need is bulk promoting.

Some other instructions

If you discipline yourself and follow the above instructions, you can gradually reduce your weight and shape your body. Besides, you have to be careful to balance immediately the diversions you may be having from this lifestyle. For example, if you manage to lose one kilo in three months with your changed lifestyle and regimen, it is quite possible to regain it with two days of careless eating. You have to be watchful and take the needed and specific action immediately. For example, if you happen to eat an excessively salty and fatty food in a restaurant, balance the effect immediately the next day by cutting down on salt and fat. Let your body release water. Eat plenty of fruits and include soup, rice and salads in your menu. Similarly, around festival times, if you have been eating a lot, carefully follow the regimen and enhance exercises as well.

4

Weight-reducing Ayurvedic Remedies

In *Charaka Samhita*, which was written 2600 years ago, Charaka has given a list of remedies that help reduce weight. In the beginning of this book, I have cited from Charaka Samhita about the ill effects of over-weight and obesity. It shows that this is an age-old problem but in our times, it is on a pandemic scale. It is clear from the first chapter of this section that we have all the weight enhancing evils in our modern lifestyle. Some of you may need the weight-reducing remedies besides the above-described methods to lose weight.

The remedies given below help to restore the balance of the doshas or the three principal energies of the body and of the dhatus (the resultant energy from the doshas). I have chosen only those remedies which are simple to make and the ingredients are also available in the West.

Remedies with trifala

Trifala is the combination of three Ayurvedic fruits— Amala, Harad and Baheda. The dried fruits without seeds are mixed together in equal quantities and a powder is made*. This powder can be used as such as a remedy as well as in combination with other drugs. Given below are the details of the drug preparation, dose and mode of consuming.

Trifala in water

Soak Trifala powder in about 200 ml of hot water, stir a little and keep it covered overnight. Next morning, make it hot and filter it. Drink it empty

---

* For more details of Trifala, see my book, *Programming Your Life with Ayurveda*

stomach in the morning and do not sit or lie down afterwards. Do yoga or go for a walk or just move around. Do not eat anything for at least half an hour after consuming Trifala.

Depending upon your constitution (prakriti) and state of health (vikriti), you may have evacuation several times. It is a process of purification.

Dose: For adults, the dose is 1 to 1½ teaspoon depending upon your body weight. For children, it is ¼ to ½ teaspoon depending on their age.

Trifala with honey

Take fine Trifala powder. If it is not a fine powder, pass it through a sieve. Put the powder in a bowl and slowly add honey into it while stirring. Make a paste and stir well. Cover the bowl and leave it like this for several hours and stir again. Store the preparation in tightly closed jars.

Dose: For adults, half a teaspoon two times a day. For children, the dose is ¼ teaspoon only once a day.

Trifala and Guggul preparation

Guggul is a raisin from a tree called *Commiphora mukul*. In Ayurveda, this raisin is also used in several other Ayurvedic drugs, notably for coronary thrombosis, arthritis, rheumatism, for strengthening bones and soft tissues and asthma.

Guggul is a very well known Ayurvedic drug and has acquired international fame. Besides its use in drugs, in India it is used in ceremonies. Due to its increasing demand in the international market, it is hard to get pure Guggul these days. Pure Guggul smells very nice and it burns leaving practically no ashes. The best test is to burn a piece and find out.

For preparing the drug for losing weight, take three parts of fine powder of Trifala and one part powdered Guggul. Mix these in honey as described above.

Dose: For adults, 1/3 of a teaspoon two times a day. For children, the dose is 1/8 of a teaspoon twice a day.

Barley and Amala preparation

Amala is one of the three fruits of Trifala. It is available abroad in the shops that keep Ayurvedic products. Make sure that it is not too old. Barley is available all over the world.

First of all, make an extract of barley. Take 250 gm of awn of barley and roast it in an iron pan until they almost become black. Crush them and soak them in six times its volume of water. After 24 hours, Filter this with a thick cloth and boil the water until it leaves some residue. This residue is called *Java Kshar* (barley extract). It has to be scrapped from the pan. You can also buy ready Java Kshar from Ayurvedic shops.

Mix one portions of barley extract with eight portions of fine amala powder. Mix them well and store the powder in a dry glass jar.

Dose: For adults, the dose is ¼ teaspoon a day. You can increase the dose to twice a day depending on the suitability and its effect on you. It is not recommended for children.

Caution: This preparation has a strong diuretic effect.

A seven-plant remedy

There are several other weight-reducing plants described in Ayurveda but they are hard to find outside India and you need to have knowledge of Ayurvedic pharmacology for preparing complicated remedies. I give you below one remedy which you can prepare on your own with some effort.

Ingredients:

Fenugreek seeds	50 gm
Ginger (dried)	50 gm
Amala (dried)	50 gm
Barley extract	10 gm

Long pepper	25 gm
Pomegranate peels (dried)	50 gm
Cress seeds	25 gm

Dry and powder all the ingredients. Make a fine powder by sieving. Mix honey in this powder and make the paste as described above.

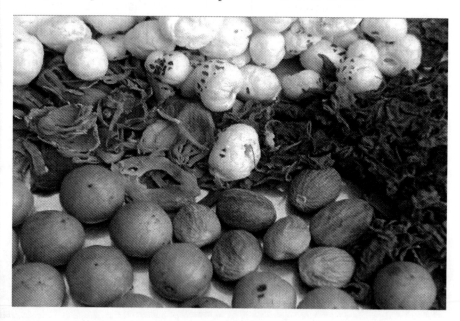

Dose: 1/3 of a teaspoon twice a day for adults and half of that dose for children.

Other Ayurvedic remedies for weight-loss

In Ayurveda, special enemas with the drugs described above are also suggested. However, you need to learn a little more about Ayurveda for using the methods of enemas on your own. There is a list of precautions to be taken before and after the enemas and they should not be applied recklessly. Lack of knowledge and care can make you sick. Therefore, I will recommend that you should not use these without proper education of Ayurveda.

Purgation is another method recommended in Ayurveda. I have described it earlier as a preparation for Ayurvedic diet and in Section III, it is recommended from time to time for maintaing weight. Enemas and purgation are a part of the purification practices of Ayurveda, called Panchkarma. They should be applied with great care and caution. See for details my book— *Programming Your Life with Ayurveda.*

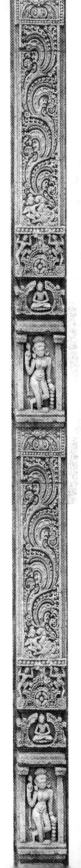

5

Losing Weight on Specific Parts of the Body

A Swiss friend of mine told me that she was 2 to 3 kg overweight and whenever she tried to lose this extra weight, she looked awful, as she first of all lost weight from her face and breasts. She would have rather liked to lose weight from her abdomen. Another friend complained that he tends to put on weight very quickly on his legs and did not know how to prevent it. There are many women who tend to put on weight on their hips. There are others who get rims of flesh on both sides of the lower back. All these persons have problems to lose weight on specific regions.

There are methods to lose weight from the specific parts of the body with special yogic exercises. That particular area where we lose weight has to reorganise with the rest. Thus, for losing weight from specific parts, we need special exercises and then for re-organisation, we also need some yoga postures or movements. With these methods, not only one loses desired weight, but also one feels rejuvenated, radiant and energetic.

Losing Weight from the hips

Generally, women have this problem more than men. Nevertheless, there are some men who by their body constitution are heavy at the back and they also tend to put on weight there.

Do following exercises to lose weight from the hips:

Exercise 1

Walking on your hips with bent knees

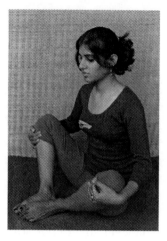

Sit down on a carpeted floor or yoga mat with bent knees. Put both your hands around each knee. Start moving forward with the movements of your hips. Your feet will move alongside but do not put pressure on them for making movements. Movements should be made by moving your hips one by one, just like you walk with your feet. After about a meter and a half, move backward in a similar manner. Moving backwards is harder and slower than moving forwards. Do this exercise for about three minutes.

Exercise 2

Walking on your hips with your feet in the air

This exercise is quite similar to the above, but it involves moving with your hips while your feet are in the air. It is much harder than the above exercise and do it only when you have successfully done the above exercise.

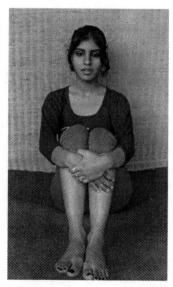

Sit in a similar manner as described above and put your arms around your bent knees. Clasp your hands together and lift your feet slightly above the ground. Your feet should touch each other. Now make movements like above exclusively with your hips. Go forward as well as backwards and do this for two minutes.

Exercise 3

Tapping with hips

Sit cross-legged and put your hands on the knees. Put all of your weight on one of your hips. Then shift the weight on the other hip. Like this do left, right, left and right hip again. It means that you have done 1,2,3, and 4. After number 4, begin again from it as number 1. That means that in the second round, you begin from the right hip where you have ended the first round. Continue like this for about 1 to 2 minutes.

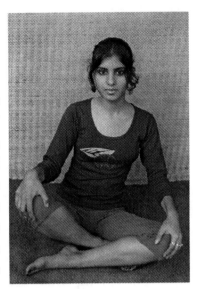

Exercise 4

Walking with your hips in cross-legged position

Sit crossed legged, rest your hands on each knee and come forward by the movements of your hips. These movements are made by shifting your weight from one hip to the other and moving forward a little the hip you have lifted. These movements are like creeping as you are almost dragging yourself on the carpet. After going forwards a little, make the backward movements. Do the exercise for 1-2 minutes.

Losing weight from legs and abdomen

The exercises given below help lose weight from the abdomen and legs. These exercises are not only good for the management of the weight but also to cure the weakness and painful conditions of the lower back and legs.

Exercise 1-4

Uttanapadasanas or the leg raising postures

There are four different asanas in this series

1. Lie down on your back with your legs nearly thirty centimetres apart from each other and arms stretched out. Make yourself at ease and let yourself loose. Gradually lift up your left leg while you inhale. Do not bend your knee in this process and the force of lifting up 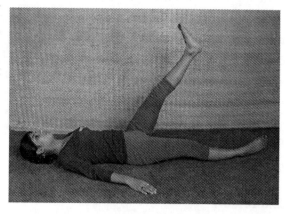 should come from your pelvic region. Lift up as much as possible without forcing yourself. Hold your breath and keep the leg still in the upward position for a few seconds. Bring the leg down gradually while exhaling. Rest for two or three breaths and then repeat the same with your right leg. Repeat this exercise for about ten times.

2: This exercise involves lifting both the legs together. Lie down on your back and put your feet together. The rest of the process is the same except that you are lifting both your legs with the feet joined together. Co-ordinate the breathing in a similar manner as described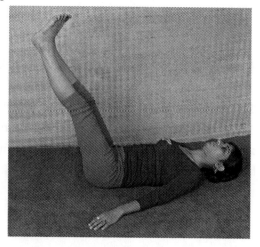

above. Repeat the exercise for about 10 times.

3,4: These exercises are done in a similar manner as above but by lying down on your stomach.

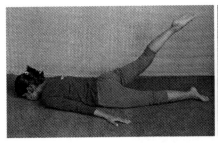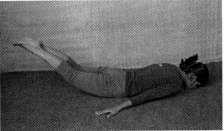

Exercise 5

Uttanapada yogabhyasa or the raised legs yogic exercises

Lie down on your back and put your legs about 30 cm apart from each other. Raise one leg like the uttanpadasana. While this leg is in the air, raise also the other leg a little. Move very slowly both the legs up and down . Do

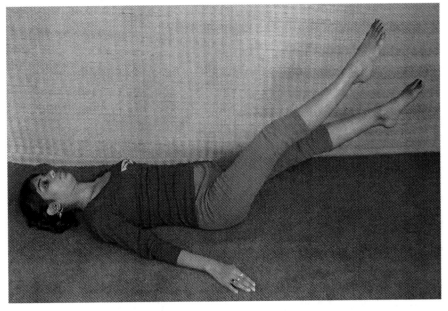

it a few times and then bring both the legs down and rest a little. This exercise is quite strenuous and learn it gradually. Do not overdo as you may get cramps in the abdomen. Your abdominal muscles will gradually get used to these movements.

Exercise 6-8

Uttanpada and rubbing the floor

Raise one of your legs as in uttanapadasana. Bend your knee and bring the foot towards the floor in such a way as if you are going to rest it there. But

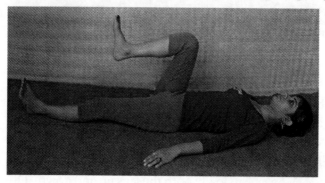

do not touch the floor with your sole. Keep the foot just above the ground. Move your foot forward in such a way as if you are rubbing your sole on the ground

but not touching it. At some point, your leg will straighten again. Raise the leg again and repeat all these movements. Do three times with one leg and three times with the other leg.

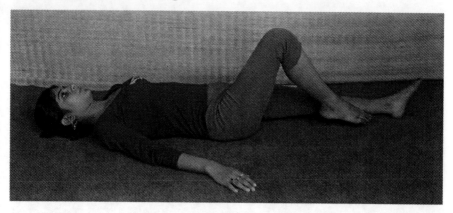

Do the next exercise with both the legs joined together. Lift them together, and bend and drag the feet in a similar manner as described above.

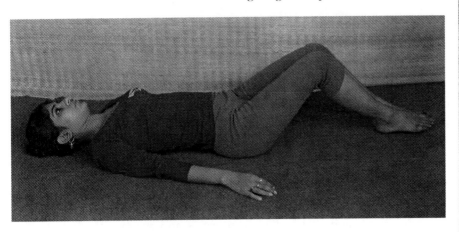

For the third exercise of this series, bend your knees, lift your feet slightly above the ground and do the rubbing of the ground (without touching the ground of course) in such a way that the movements of your feet are in the opposite direction from each other.

Exercise 9, 10

Kicking while lying down

Lie down on your back and fold your right leg in such a way that your thigh is almost touching your abdomen and the foot is straight. Kick in the air. Repeat the same with the left leg. Do the exercise at least five times by alternating the legs.

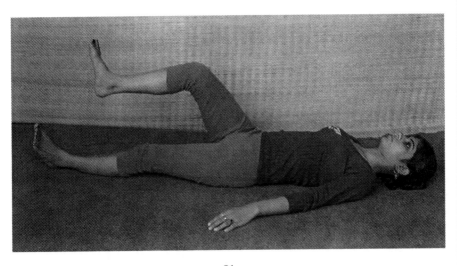

The next exercise is to do the kicking in the same manner as above but with both the legs together. Lie down as described above but join your legs and feet. Fold your legs and do similar kicking as above with both the legs together while the feet remain joined.

Exercise 11

This exercise is from breathing practices of yoga— the pranayama. Sit down in a comfortable posture, preferably cross-legged. Take a deep breath slowly while pulling in the abdominal muscles simultaneously. Hold for a brief moment the pulled in muscles and the breath. Release the breath as well as the abdominal muscles gradually and simultaneously. Repeat this practice 10-15 times in the morning and before going to bed at night. This practice is called *dhaunkni*. Dhaunkni is a small leather pouch with a pressing handle used to blow air for lighting the firewood.

Suggestion: You can do this several times a day and also while at work. Do not do that until two hours after the main meals.

Losing weight from thoracic region and chin

Many people get a persistent rim of flesh in their thoracic region. It bulges out even more after having eaten. Besides the excessive fat in this area, they often have a problem with their agni or digestive fire. Do the exercises given below regularly to get rid of the thoracic flesh rim and you will also benefit from them to get a better digestion and assimilation of food. These exercises stretch your chin muscles as well thus taking care of the problem of double chin.

Exercise 1

Bhujangasana or the cobra posture

1. In this asana, you will lift up your head and chest while lying down on the stomach. Lie down on your stomach and let your chin rest on the floor. Put your hands nearly at the level of your chest and your arms will bend in this

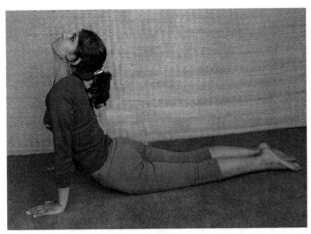

process. Now lift your head and chest gradually while inhaling. Bend as far back as you comfortably can and straighten your arms. Stay only for few seconds in this posture and your breath should be held inside during this time. Bring gradually your head and chest downwards while exhaling. Repeat the asana 4-5 times.

Exercise 2

Bhujang-uttanasana or the cobra posture with raised leg

Lie down on your stomach as described above. Lift up your head and chest and one of the legs simultaneously. By keeping a gap of few breaths, repeat the asana with the other leg. Enhance the duration of the asana by regular practice. Repeat 4-5 times.

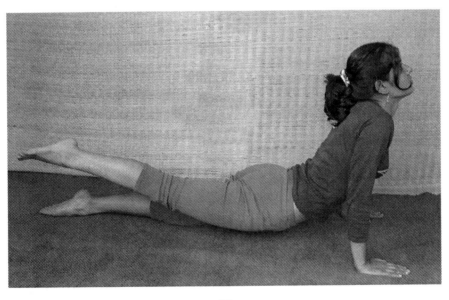

Exercise 3

Dhanurasana or bow posture

Lie down on your stomach. Bend your legs from the knees and bring your ankles as close to your hips as possible. Stretch back your arms and hold

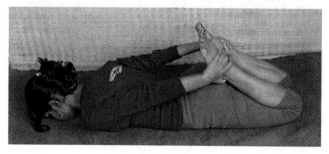

your ankles with your hand. Tighten the grip and lift up your body by applying force from the hands and arms. Your body makes the shape of a bow in this asana. Never go beyond your capacity and stay

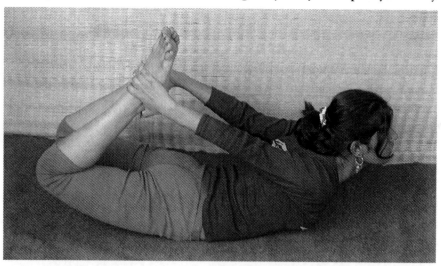

for a short while in this asana specially in the beginning. Repeat 2-3 times.

The above two asanas energise all the internal organs of the body, muscles and joints besides trimming the extra flesh from your thoracic region.

Exercise 4

Ustrasana or Camel posture

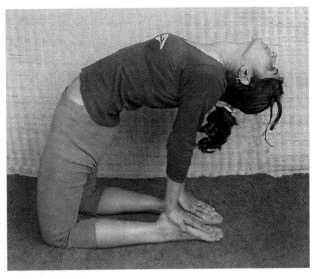

Sit on your knees with the legs bent backwards. In fact, it is like half standing on your knees. Stretch your arms backwards and also bend your body backwards and touch your feet with your hands as shown in Figure.

Losing weight from lower back

Some people tend to put on extra flesh on both sides of the lower back. Uttanapadasanas described above for the abdomen also help to reduce the weight on the lower back. Here are some more exercises which will help to reduce fat accumulation on this part of the body.

Exercise 1-2

Circular movements with the foreleg

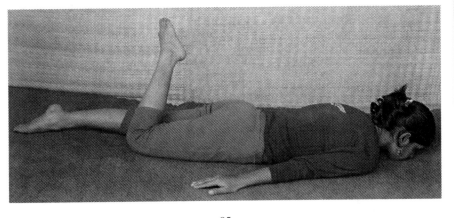

Lie down on your stomach. Bend your leg from the knee in such a way that your foreleg is in a vertical position. Make clockwise round movements with this portion of your leg. It is like you are making circles in the air with your foot. Make five circles and then alternate the leg to repeat the same. Rest for five breaths and repeat the exercise but making anticlockwise movements this time.

The next exercise is to make the circular movements in both directions but this time with both the legs together. Lie down on your stomach, join your feet together and bend your legs from the knees. Make the circular movements as described above. Remember to make the movements at 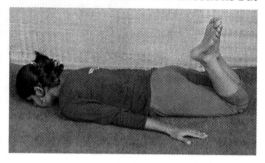 least five times clockwise and another five times anticlockwise.

Exercise 3, 4

Upward and sideways stretching of the legs

Lie down on your back. Bring yourself to a completely relaxed posture. Lift your left leg upwards like you did in Uttanpadasana. Bring the raised

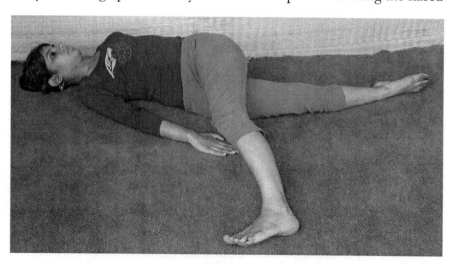

left leg towards the right direction and touch the ground with your foot. Stay in this posture as long as you comfortably can and then bring the leg back slowly in the straight position. After a rest of few breaths, repeat the same for the right leg. Do the exercise at least five times.

The next exercise is similar but is done while lying on the stomach. In this position, the leg cannot be stretched out straight without bending the knee. Repeat the exercise for at least five times.

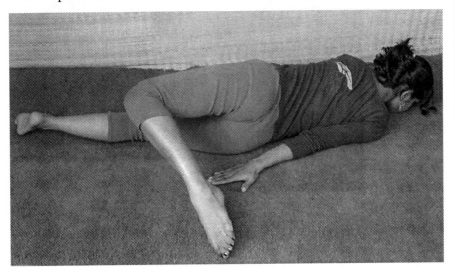

Losing weight from the waist

The exercises for abdomen evidently will trim your waist but women wish to have an extra curve at this place. To get rid of excess fat from the waist and enhance the curve, here are some simple exercises.

Exercise 1

Waist tilting

Sit down on your heels and stretch your arms upwards. Clasp both your hands together by intertwining your fingers. Palms of your hands should be facing upwards and the arms should be straight. Tilt yourself from your waist towards left and stay in this position for a little while. Return to the straight posture again, relax and then tilt towards the right side from your waist. Make sure that the rest of your body stays straight. Otherwise the pressure will not be focussed on the waist.

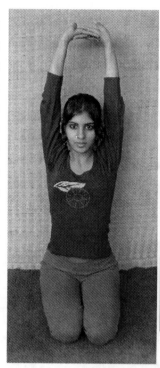
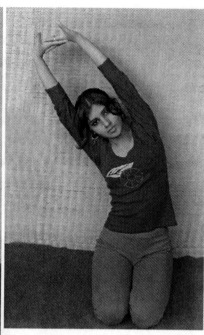

Exercise 2

Round movements with waist

Stand straight, let yourself loose and put both your arms upwards. Clasp both your hands together and turn the palms upwards. Make round movements clockwise by moving your waist in circles. Make sure that your head stays between both your arms and your movements are very slow. Make 3 to 5 movements. Rest for 2-3 breaths and make the same number of movements anticlockwise

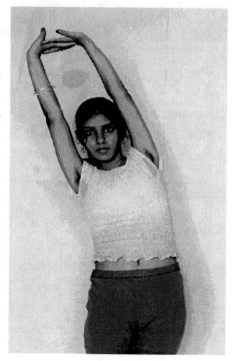

Exercise 3

Waist twisting

Bend forward, clasp both your hands together with the palms facing downwards. Stay like this for a little while and then move on your left side from the waist in such a way that your clasped hands are almost on the side of your left leg. Do the same for the right side. Repeat at least five times.

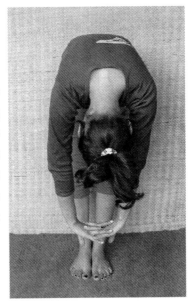

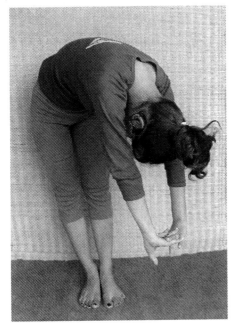

Other than the exercise described above, Yoga nritya (yoga dance) will be very beneficial to trim the waist. Refer to my book— *The Natural Glamour.*

6

Balancing the Space and Fire Elements

Interrelationship of the five elements, which constitute the whole cosmos including our body, is very important in Ayurveda. The balance of the five elements signifies health and their disproportion leads to disorders and malfunctions. Excess weight is also a malfunction due to some imbalance. The holistic way of looking at the cosmos and the body is very subtle and we cannot simply state that the solid structure of the body is constituted of kapha (water and earth elements), therefore overweight is a problem of the imbalance of kapha. It is not basically a false statement but it is too simplistic as the interaction of the water and the earth are not independent of the other three elements. Let me give a mundane example to make you understand the interaction. If you have a wet piece of cloth and you want to dry it quickly, the simple method is to spread it and move it around in the air. Thus, the element space and air have a drying effect. Similarly, heat has a drying effect. In the following pages, you will learn that how the elements space and fire are important in concrete and subtle ways to the problem of excessive body weight. Overweight and obesity are due to the disorder of dhatus and not exclusively a kapha imbalance as is understood by many abroad after having gained a little knowledge of Ayurveda. The food we eat should contribute to the formation of eight principal dhatus or accumulative energies of the body. Due to a disorder, certain persons accumulate fat dhatu in excess and not the other dhatus.

Transformation of food into dhatus is the principal function of the digestive fire or agni. The distribution of the principal dhatu (rasa dhatu) into other dhatus is the function of vata (air and space elements). Thus, for bringing the body to balance so that it does not accumulate exclusively the fat dhatu, a subtle understanding of our dynamic body in this dynamic cosmos is essential.

Space

It is not enough to do exercises to lose weight within a limited space. According to Vedic wisdom, the element space or ether, called aakasha in Sanskrit, is the first fundamental element of the five elements which constitute the cosmos. In fact, this is the primary element, as without space, nothing can exist. In space is air, which provides us prana or the living element through our breathing process. The fire can exist only with space and air. Water can exist when space, air and fire are present. Without the heat of the fire, the water will solidify as was during the Ice Age. The fifth element earth consists of all the previous four elements and is the heaviest of all.

According to Ayurveda, everything in the cosmos is constituted of these five elements and so is the human body. In all living beings, the five elements take the form of the three principal energies or vital forces (vata, pitta, kapha), which perform all the physical and mental functions of the body. The equilibrium of these three energies signifies health and their imbalance causes discomfort, ailments and disorders. Being overweight is a problem of the element space. It is the expansion of the inner space in terms of the physical mass of the body.

In order to acquire harmony and balance and get back to the perfect shape of the body, it is not merely the so-called 'workouts' which count. You need to expand yourself in the outer space in order to harmonise your inner space. In other words, it is essential that you include long walks and outings to balance the space element in your body.

To put this idea in practice, I recommend that you go for a walk at least 10 minutes after your two main meals. On your day off or Sunday, take a longer walk. Many housewives put on weight despite doing lots of housework and going up and down due to their activities in a limited space. Make it a point to go out everyday in a disciplined manner. Get into the habit of stretching your body as much as you can. Those of you who have learnt yogasanas probably know the art of expanding and shrinking the body in space.

In brief, make an effort to expand your body in space and give yourself the privilege of roaming in the open spaces in the cosmos. A trekker can best relate to the experience of the cosmic space. To breathe the air in the high mountains of the Himalayas is an intake of the element space from the cosmos. According to yoga, the air we breathe is prana or life. That is what keeps body and soul together. The quality of pranic energy varies from place to place. Compare the energy you are taking inside you in the mountains to the tiny closed room somewhere in the city. Your body and the breathing mechanism is the same, but the quality of prana is different and therefore your cosmic connection is different in these two places.

This concept may sound bizarre to some of you but remember that Ayurveda does not treat the body and the cosmos like a machine. Cosmos is a dynamic whole where everything is interrelated, interconnected and interdependent. There is oneness in nature and the same principles are applicable on human body as on cosmos. Thus, there are many subtle relationships between all what exist and these cannot be measured or recorded by existing machines.

Digestive fire or Agni

Vitiation and imbalance in the digestive fire leads to the vitiation of dhatus and thus may give rise to the problem of overweight. Therefore, take care of your fire element so that the digestive fire works well and does not disturb the balance of the dhatus. If the digestive fire is in equilibrium, you have a balance between rasa (essence of the food the body assimilates) and *mala* (that which is eliminated in the form of faeces, urine, sweat, etc.). This balance is very important for maintaining the right weight. Persons with disturbed agni sometimes eat a lot and eliminate very little. Therefore they put on weight very easily.

Another symptom of agni imbalance is excessive hunger. Obviously it leads to excess of weight. Generally persons with vata disturbance have their agni sometimes low and sometimes high. It is just like the wind makes a flame quiver low and high. Thus, there are phases of excessive hunger which lead to overweight in these individuals.

If you have a normal agni, you will be quite regular in your meal times and the quantity of food you consume. If your agni is disturbed, you will get false hunger alarms leading to excess weight. However, lack of appetite is also due to disturbed agni. In any case, if you have any symptoms of disturbed agni, you should make every effort to acquire an equilibrium.

To create an equilibrium of agni, you need the purgation treatment. Purgation purifies the digestive fire and balances it. Take care to observe all the precautions described before and after the treatment of purgation.

After purgation, begin with a simple and warm liquid diet and gradually increase the diet. Eat the meals on time and be careful about the quantity and quality of food you consume. If your stomach is sensitive, take bitter teas like wormwood or neem mixed with ajwain and ginger.

Long sitting sessions, specially those which involve doing desk work can also vitiate agni. Therefore, be careful about your posture. Try to keep a footrest and break the long sitting sessions with some stretching exercises and movements.

If you often have problems of acidity and other stomach and liver related problems and they do not go away with the purgation therapy, consult a physician.

7

Psychological Aspects of over-weight

Mental conflicts and crisis can lead to excess weight in some cases. The root cause for this is *asantosha* or a mental state of dissatisfaction. Due to lack of wisdom, many people live in a state of asantosha. It is the lack of control on the activities of one's mind. The mental state of dissatisfaction leads one to seek different ways of fulfilment. Some persons take to eating excessively; there are others who buy too many shoes or clothes. There are still others who join strange sects or groups to find their fulfilment.

Excessive eating due to frustration

Let us see what are the possible factors, which generally cause dissatisfaction and make people frustrated.

- ☐ Lack of sex
- ☐ Frustration with children or family in general
- ☐ Problems at work-place
- ☐ Problems in social life
- ☐ Feeling of failure in one's own life

Out of frustration, many people take to excessive eating. They yearn to eat something even after a full meal. They tend to eat specially in the evening when they are at home. Those ones who stay at home or work at home may do the same after lunch or other times of the day. In this process, they not only put on extra weight but also ruin their digestive system. This kind of behaviour is different from the other when people simply eat too much for meals. This latter category of people eat out of greed and satisfaction of their senses. They usually eat too much only when the food is good. They look for good restaurants and chose those places for holidays where good meals are offered. These ones have sensuous fulfilment in eating big meals in large quantity. But at present we are talking of those who eat due to a sense of dissatisfaction and frustration. They eat anything or everything and tend to eat junk food.

Solutions: My purpose to write this chapter is not to provide you psychotherapy but to make you aware so that you are able to analyse yourself and work on yourself. The best way is to face the real issue and to deal with it. If something is missing in your life or is not according to your desire and wishes, there are two ways to handle it. Either you change your life or accept the situation with a smile. Most people find themselves in the state of frustration because they neither accept the circumstances they are in, nor do they make an effort to get out of it. In fact, they grumble and overlook the positive aspects of their situation. A decision to change is hard for them as they lack courage and do not want to leave the comfort and assurance their present situation provides them.

If you fall in this category, the ultimate solution to control weight lies in going to the root of the problem and solve it. Even if you manage to lose weight by following the diet and other instructions in this book, the problem can recur. What you really need in such cases is first of all to quieten your mind. To do it, you need to be alone and away from the family. Do some breathing exercises, go for long walks and then think about your irrationality of putting your frustrations down in your alimentary canal in the form of food. If you really feel that you are suffering due to whatever reason, this act of pacifying yourself with food will actually enhance your troubles by making you ill in the long run. Thus, think of the real issue and face it. Be strict with yourself to refrain from eating except at meal times. This will help to bring the subdued emotions on surface.

Shifting responsibility

Many people give false reasons for their bulky body and shirk from the responsibility of doing something for themselves. Often they blame it on others in the family, like 'my husband or wife or child eats too much sweet or other junk food or fried stuff' and so on. There are many women who blame their overweight and deformed figure on childbirth. If you acquire this attitude of blaming others or specific situations, you do not take any responsibility for yourself. In that case you let things happen and find a way to escape from the real issue. Each one of us is responsible for herself/himself. If due to overweight, you become prey to disorders, it will affect your family as well but none will suffer as you will do. Therefore, take your own responsibility and do something to change your attitude and lifestyle.

Many a times, I see entire families of three or four members overweight. Besides the lifestyle error, there are emotional factors in such cases which lead to the mismanagement of the family. For example, parents need to spend time to train children to distinguish between nourishment and junk food. Many parents do not do that because of their preoccupation with their own problems at work or with each other. Children, on the other hand, feel very lonely in such cases and due to that they take to excessive and untimely eating habits.

Solution: Remember the aphorism from Ayurveda that the first priority of life is life itself. Food is the fundamental factor for our health and longevity. Ailment or death brings end to life. Thus, you as a family or an individual should treat food with sanctity and it should be on your priority list. It should not be sidelined by ordering food from restaurants and going out often. Good quality food, prepared with love, eaten ceremoniously with a good mental state and in a good atmosphere can change your life, relationships and way of thinking.

Section II
Some Specific
Factors for
Weight-loss

1

Combination of Various Practices for Achieving a Specific Goal

In Section I of the book, I have provided you the general Ayurvedic wisdom to lose weight. There are some aspects of the weight loss that you should always follow. For example, you should be aware of the weight-enhancing factors and should try your best to avoid them. On the other hand, all of you may not need the remedies for losing weight. However, persons with excessive overweight may need a very specific diet as well as remedies. For optimum results from the wisdom provided in this book, you are required to learn to use various precautions and methods for losing weight according to the need and situation.

In this chapter, I will provide you with the guidelines to integrate different methods to lose weight for a specific aim. This will give you a more efficient way to lose weight on some specific parts of your body with the combination of diverse methods. It is essential that you learn to use the wisdom provided in this book in an integrated way for getting not only the right weight on your scale but also to have a beautiful form of your body. At times, you experience that although you have not gained any extra kilo on the scale but nevertheless, you look fatter than before on certain part of your body. This happens usually on the abdominal area. Besides that, in some cases, the excessive weight also leads to fat accumulation in the form of nodules and it is very essential to get rid of them. Such fat-knots block the flow of energy and may lead to certain disorder.

Balancing weight on abdominal area

Putting weight on the abdominal area is a most usual problem of both men and women all over the world. Men usually develop paunch and women have two different zones in upper and lower abdomen that bulge out. I have many interesting explanations from various people about their paunch or abdominal rings. 'Beer-belly' is the most common expression in Germany that is used for explaining the reason for a paunch. A friend of mine called his paunch as 'computer belly', signifying thereby that it is due to sitting for long hours in front of the computer. Most women tend to attribute their abdominal fat rings to childbirth. Whatever your explanations may be, my aim is to teach you the efficient ways to shape your body.

Beer or computer or childbirth contributes to the abdominal fat due to a lack of balance of these activities to your lifestyle and food habits. Beer may give rise to vata imbalance in the lower abdomen and cause wind. But beer is really not directly responsible for the paunch Pretzels eaten with beer may be. Principally, along with beer, it is the cold dinner with lot of cheese and meat and followed by sitting rather than going for a walk is responsible for the abdominal fat in Germany. If you do not wish to give up beer, try to make the following changes in your lifestyle in order to avoid the paunch.

☐ Drink only a very small portion of beer with your dinner or preferably none at all. Take your beer one hour after dinner. Beverages containing alcohol are not recommended before dinner, when your stomach is empty. In case you absolutely want to drink beer before meal, then take it one hour before your meal with very light snack and not something heavy which is made of wheat or other grains. For example, take nuts in a very small quantity. However, I do not suggest this method as a priority. I highly recommend not drinking beer or any other alcoholic beverage before dinner.

☐ Take a vegetable or chicken soup for dinner along with a salad. Avoid bread and if you need something substantial, take boiled potatoes. Alternatively, take a plate of fresh vegetables along with some cheese or small pieces of chicken. Do not take cheese and meat together. Do not take any other meet. Cook your meals in very little quantity of olive or sesames and not with butter or ghee. The principal objective here is to reduce the intake of fat in general and to minimise the consumption of animal fat.

☐ Include in your meals plenty of fresh ginger, pepper, ajwain and cumin. These spices will treat your vata imbalance caused due to beer. They will prevent the accumulation of wind in the abdomen.

☐ Eat your dinner at least two hours before going to bed and do not sit immediately after dinner. Go for a walk for at least 15 minutes, preferably for half an hour.

☐ Do the yogic exercises described for reducing the excessive flesh around the abdominal area (see Section I, Chapter 6)

Those of you who accumulate fat around the abdominal area due to long hours of deskwork should pay attention to the following:

☐ Break the sitting sessions by getting up in between and doing some stretching exercises. If you cannot afford to get up, get use to doing movements with your feet and waist while you are sitting. Stretch up your arms, hold your hands together and make circular movements with them. Put your both hands behind your neck and clasp them. . Your hands should not touch your head but should stay apart. While in this position, twist your waist to extreme left and then to extreme right.

☐ Take care to reduce the animal fat intake (meat, butter or ghee, milk, cheese). You should not completely leave out the animal fat as its deficiency leads to vata imbalance. But keep in mind that the accumulation of fat specifically on this portion enhances very quickly with excess of animal fat.

☐ Balance your long sitting hours with an after dinner walk. Some people get kapha vikriti due to jobs that involve sitting for a long time and they develop and inertia. In the evening at home, they end up sitting again. Keep a vigil on yourself and balance your work situation with activity and long walks.

Accumulation of Adipose tissue

Accumulation of fat nodules in the legs or elsewhere is another problem in some cases of overweight. One should pay immediate attention to this problem as the accumulation of adipose tissue blocks srotas or the energy channels and leads to various ailments. Given below are some suggestions to get rid of this problem.

☐ Be very strict with your diet and follow the diet plan described in the previous section.

☐ In addition to the diet, you need to do yogic exercises as well as morning and evening walk. I suggest that you do everyday 12 times the yogic exercises of Surya Namaskar or prostration to the sun.

☐ Take baths regularly with some essential oils in your bath. Stay in the bath until you begin to perspire.

☐ Application of wet heat is essential on the area where there is fat accumulation. This is done with wet towels in hot water containing a combination of pain-relieving essential oils.

2

Protection of the Body during Weight-loss

A pregnant woman gets stretch marks if she does not take appropriate care during her pregnancy. With increase in weight, the outer skin stretches just like the abdomen during pregnancy. Perhaps you have observed people who succeed in losing weight quite rapidly begin to look old and haggard and acquire a 'drained out' appearance. This chapter provides you the essential instructions to take care of the skin so that you do not get loose skin, stretch marks or tissue drainage during the process of losing weight.

To save the outer appearance of the body from any damage during the process of losing weight, there are two principal things you should do regularly:

☐ Anoint the body with oil or other products with fat (snehan) everyday or every other day.

☐ Do yogic exercises or stretching exercises given in this book regularly.

Fat application on the skin

Snehan* as it is called in Ayurveda, is the treatment of the body with oils, ghee or some mixtures like ghee, oil, milk, cream, honey etc. This treatment strengthens the skin, provides it more elasticity and makes the body stronger. It saves the skin from external infections as well. In the present context, our aim is to enhance the elasticity of the skin so that it

---

* Another meaning of snehan is affection. Treatment of body with tender and unctuous substances provides protection and strength to the body and solace to the mind

can adjust to the decline in the volume of the body. You can follow one or more of the methods given below:

☐ The most simple and the least time consuming method for oil application is that you apply warm coconut, olive or sesame oil all over your body immediately after bathing or showering with warm or hot water. Take some oil on your palm and apply on your skin with some force. Apply on all parts of the body, paying special attention to areas which are more fleshy. For example, give extra strokes and rub oil several times on hips, thighs and abdomen. These are the areas susceptible to get tissue drainage and stretch marks in the process of losing weight. The body absorbs the oils after rubbing several times. In the end, wash yourself with warm water to take off the extra oil from the skin.

☐ If you have a very dry skin, you need to do an oil saturation self-massage twice a week. Sit down comfortably in a warm place. Rub one of the above-stated warm oils on your body in a systematic manner. Massage your left hand and arm with the right hand and

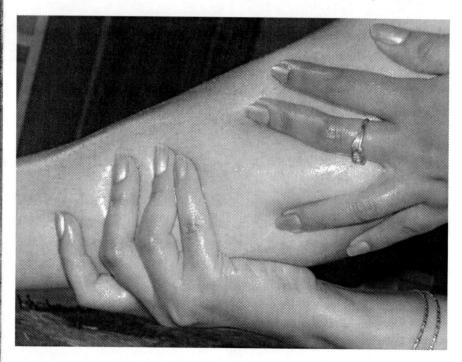

then the other way around. Apply smooth pressure and make several strokes. Then do your feet and legs one after the other by using some force with both your hands. Do long strokes of massage with force. Rub the oil on the abdomen, chest and neck. Massage your shoulders and back of the neck. If the body has absorbed all the oil you have applied, repeat the process. In the end, make a hand towel wet in hot water, squeeze it and wipe off the superfluous oil. Do not take a shower immediately after this treatment. Leave the oil on your body for several hours or overnight.

☐ Give yourself a treatment of gods with the following mixture:

Add the following in equal quantities and whip them together:

a. Honey
b. Sesame or olive oil
c. Milk cream
d. Ghee

After whipping, this mixture will become like a cream and can be stored in the refrigerator for several days. Apply this on your dry body after your shower. Rub well everywhere and wash off the superfluous fat with hot water. This mixture makes the skin smooth like a baby.

Physical activities

Make an effort to stay active so that along with the oil application, your body muscles get a regular exercise. The oil application is to take care of the outer part of the body and activities with yoga, stretching and going for walks are to reach deeper and activate your muscles, joints and internal organs.

Based upon Ayurvedic principles, I am describing the holistic way of dealing with your body and involve each and every part of your being in the process of losing weight. Feel mentally involved with the process of trimming and reshaping yourself. Tell your self to avoid long sitting sessions and take thirty seconds to stretch yourself in diverse directions after every hour.

Take time to do yogic exercises given in this book. They will help to shape you properly and enhance your beauty during weight loss. Make sure also to take a walk, specially after dinner. Even if you cannot go out due to bad weather or some other reason, walk for about ten minutes inside the house or else involve yourself with the activities which demand your movements.

Those of you, who have learnt dancing of some kind, can use this mode of activity so that the weight-loss is not a passive process that gives you wrinkles but an active process that rejuvenates you.

3

Practices for Excessive Overweight

Let us define first of all what we mean by over-weight and what is excessive over-weight or obesity that I am going to consider in this chapter. Maximum of up to 25 % of the normal weight of a person can be considered as over-weight whereas above that percentage, a person may be considered as obese. It is not possible to get a definite formula for so-called normal weight. It is more the shape and form of the body that should be taken into consideration. Two persons of the same height and age may have different weight but none of them may be over-weight. The difference in weight can also be due to the variation in muscular and bone structures of these two individuals. In Ayurveda, such diversity in body weight is designated to the difference in proportion of the diverse *dhatus*. Dhatus are the resultant material of the three energies of the body (vata, pitta and kapha). They form the supporting system of the body. There are seven principal dhatus. These are: rasa (essence of nutrition), rakta (blood), mansa (muscles), meda (adipose tissue or fat), asthi (bone), manja (bone marrow) and shukra (sexual excretions).

In a Science dictionary, obesity is defined as follows:

The condition of a person having excessive weight for his height, built and age because of a build up of fat. Obesity is common in western society. It predisposes to or is associated with numerous diseases including diabetes, arthritis, arteriosclerosis and high blood pressure.

This, however, is a rather non-specific description of obesity.

It is worth noting that rarely, obesity is due to pathological reasons and you need to get medical examination in such cases in order to take the appropriate treatment. It is estimated that only 5% cases of obesity may be due to hormonal imbalance, thyroid problems or other pathological conditions in the body. Obesity should not be confused with oedema. Oedema is due to water retention in the body.

It is important to understand that there are several other features that distinguish obesity from over-weight and that even 20 to 25% of excessive weight from the usual weight of a person may be classified as obesity in certain cases. Nodules of the adipose tissue and fat formation under the skin, loose flesh and excessively disproportionate body are the signs of obesity. However, there are persons with same percentage of excessive weight but due to physical activity, they are not flabby. These persons need several measures simultaneously to get rid of their excessive weight described in the previous section. The other ones with more predominant signs of obesity as described here will have to go through a more rigorous diet and exercise to get the situation in control. I will describe below some diet and exercise programme for persons suffering from excessive over-weight or obesity. Needless to say that you require tremendous effort, mental discipline and persistence to achieve success but always think that it is better than being ill and suffer, or cut short one's lifespan.

It is logical that if the problem of overweight is grave, one has to make rigorous efforts to bring it down. The other part is that heavier a person is, more inertia exists in making an effort to get rid of the extra weight. In fact, excessive over-weight leads to imbalance of kapha, which ultimately gives rise to inertia. Therefore, in several cases of obesity, an appropriate counselling is required to initiate an individual for making a rigorous effort for getting rid of extra weight and reshaping the body.

Plan of action for reducing excessive weight

Here is a five-fold plan of action for fighting against obesity:

1   Yogic concentration practices and breathing exercises (pranayama) to gain mental strength and to enhance determination for achievement of the goal.

2. Treatment with wet heat.

3. A very strict diet plan.

4. Walks and other bodily movements in a very disciplined manner.

5. Trifala treatment to reduce weight and regain body's equilibrium.

Yogic practices

Here are three different yogic steps to make you more conscious of your excessive weight and provide you courage and determination to fight back against obesity. These methods will evoke sattva (peace and stillness of mind) in you, which will help you get rid of your inertia and will initiate you to be healthy and to attain a good body shape.

☐ **Visualising your body:** Imagine the form of your body. Sit down in a relaxed posture and let yourself loose. The important part is to develop the ability to be able to sit still for a while. Once you have a relaxed and still posture, close your eyes, concentrate on your breathing and let the energy of your breath flow in all parts of your body. Imagine the space your body occupies. With each breath, repeat in your mind- 'I am going to reshape my body'. Do that for about 10 times. Gradually open your eyes and get ready for the next step.

☐ **Pressing your body:** This step involves pressing your body. Press all parts of your body in a systematic manner. Begin pressing your left hand and arm with the right hand. Press each place with strong grip and several times. After this, press right hand and arm with the left hand in a similar manner. Now press the left feet and leg with both the hands. Similarly, press the right feet and leg. Press front part of the body with both your hands. Press your shoulders with both your hands and press your back as far as you can reach it.

☐ **Pranayama or the breathing exercises:** This is a programme with 25 breaths. You are supposed to send your breath to a particular part of the body. I have described below the yogic names and places for these breaths. Do each type of breathing five times in a row.

1. Prana in technical language of Patanjali means breathing for the plexus region. Bring your breath to the chest region or the region of your plexus.

2. Samana literally means equal and in the technical language of yoga, it denotes the middle of the body, a point that divides the body into two equal halves: upper and lower. Bring your breath to your navel.

3. Apana means lower or lower part of the body. For the third breath, bring your breath between the navel region and your feet and send the vital air to this area.

4.Udana means upper or rising. The breath is sent to the head region.

5. Vyana means one of the three vital forces of the body, called vata. This vital force, like the element air and ether it comes from, is everywhere in the body, thus the breath is sent to all parts of the body.

While doing Udana, repeat in your mind- 'I am going to be lighter and slimmer'.

While doing Vyana, repeat the following: 'I am going to be strong and healthy from lose and flabby'.

Wet heat treatment

In Ayurveda, the heat treatment is called fomentation or perspiration therapy and it is two kinds⁻ dry and wet. Dry consists of sweating in dry and hot place (like a sauna) and wet is like a vapour bath. However, in Ayurveda, exposing to cold or air is strictly forbidden after fomentation therapy. I describe below a simple method to do wet fomentation at home with a specific bath.

☐   Before your bath, make sure that you close all the windows and the place should be warm. Prepare your bed and make it warm with a hot water bottle. Make some ginger + basil + cardamom + pepper tea in a thermos and keep it besides your bed.

☐ Prepare a hot bath. Add some drops of essential oils like rose, jasmine, fennel and Eucalyptus into it. Sit in the bath comfortably and make sure that the water remains hot. Add more hot water from time to time.

☐ When you start sweating, come out of your bath, put on a bathrobe and go to your warm bed. Take some tea and rest fully covered. You will continue to sweat for a while.

☐ Rest for at least ½ an hour after you have stopped sweating.

Alternatively, you can do the wet heat treatment with hot towels. Heat water in a big pot and put some essential oils in it. Put small towels into it. Squeeze the towels with the help of a forceps and lay them on your body taking care that they are not too hot. You have to constantly heat the water for changing the towels. Do it for about 20 minutes and then take rest as described above. This treatment is particularly beneficial for getting rid of the fat nodules. You may do this treatment only on some specific parts of the body to get rid of the adipose accumulation.

Diet plan

Unlike the diet plan in the last section where I have described fine recipes, this rigorous diet is mainly meant for survival so that you can initiate the process of losing weight and gaining shape and strength. However, after about five weeks of this diet, you can introduce some recipes from the previous section, taking care to consume very little salt and doing strictly the low fat cooking as has been described.

Breakfast

After your early morning hot water and exercises, leave as much time as you possibly can to take breakfast. Take rejuvenating tea and for breakfast eat only fruits but not bananas. Eat sweet fruits like dates, papaya, sweet raisins or sweet apples. You may cook the apples if you want warm food. Alternatively, if you are able to obtain two products abroad, they can make a very nice breakfast without adding up fat to you. These are Phool makhana and Seel. Phool makhana is made from a lotus like plant by heating its anterior fluid. They are white, round balls, little bigger than a cherry in size. They are available at the Indian shops abroad. Seel looks like a grain but it is not. It is nearly white in colour and the grains are smaller than mustard seeds.

Recipe for Phool Makhana

Roast them on a hot iron pan for few minutes to make them crisp. Powder them in a grinder. Take 3-4 tablespoons of this powder with 100 ml of hot milk*.

Recipe for Seel

Seel grains have to be roasted in a hot pan by stirring constantly. The grains become puffed and light with heat. Take 4-5 tablespoons of puffed grains of Seel in 100 ml of hot milk.

Main meals

Main meals should contain chapati or roti of the roasted grains of barley or wheat. Barley is bulk decreasing and should be preferred. You can also make a kind of bread with the flour of the roasted grains if you find chapatti making cumbersome. Recipe for chapati or roti is given in Chapter 2 of Section I. The bread or chapatti should be accompanied by some preparation of the green vegetables. You may make mixed vegetables from time to time but at least once a day, you should take green vegetable. Use of Stinging Nettle is highly recommended as it is bulk decreasing. Take carrot, turnip or tomato or some similar vegetables as salad but these should be slightly steamed with a spoon of water in them and in a tightly closed pan. It is a warm salad. Add a little lemon juice and

---

* In Ayurveda, we do not recommend to take fat-free milk. Products should be taken in their natural form.

half a teaspoon of olive or sesames oil into it.

For dessert, eat either 15 raisins or three dates or two figs.

Besides your diets, pay attention to the following:

- [ ] Minimize the quantity of salt, sugar and fat but do not leave any of them totally.
- [ ] Preferably, avoid using salt for dinners as green vegetables have enough of salt contents. Use exclusively rock salt*.
- [ ] Take hot water with lemon one hour after lunch. Alternatively, take water cooked with little ginger or cardamom.
- [ ] Take dinner three hours before going to bed.
- [ ] Drink some cardamom water before going to bed.
- [ ] If you feel week or feel hungry specially in the initial days of dieting, take some dried raisins. Eat them one by one.

Physical activity

Morning walk

After drinking a glass of hot water (preferably boiled with cardamom), take a walk for at least half an hour. Do not eat breakfast before going for a walk. You need to drink only hot water in order to purify your system.

Walk after meals

Make it a point never to sit down after two main meals. Even if you do not have much time after lunch, do spare at least 15 minutes to walk. Walk for an hour after dinner.

Other activities

Even if you are a desk worker, do include some movements of hands, feet

---

* Rock salt is being marketed as Himalayan salt in Europe.

and limbs which can be done easily while sitting. During the intermittent breaks from work, do some stretching exercises by pulling up the arms, bending forward and backward and so on.

Trifala treatment

Trifala treatment has already been described in Chapter 4, Section I. During this rigorous diet, take trifala treatment with water but add liquorice to Trifala in the ratio of one to four. Add 25 gm of liquorice into 75 gm of trifala and mix well. Take this remedy with water every morning as has been described in Section I, Chapter 4.

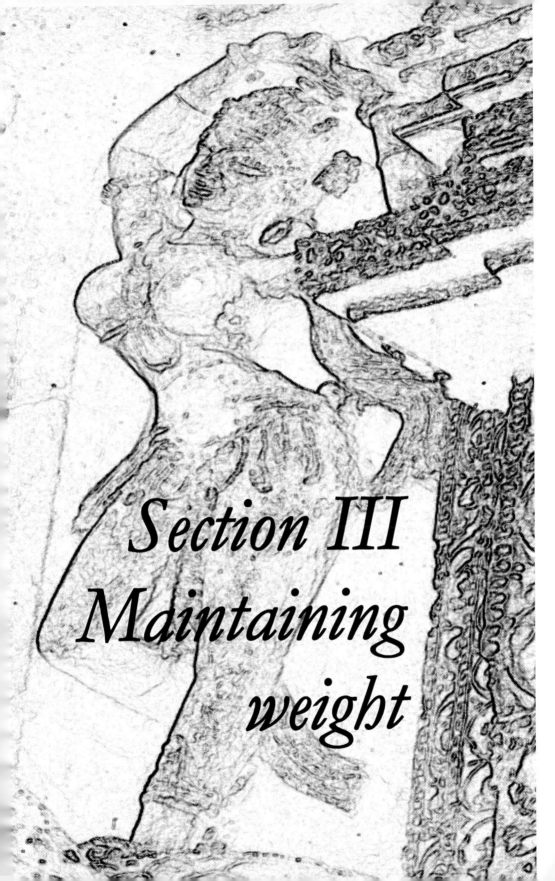

Section III
Maintaining weight

1

Healthy and Balanced Ayurvedic Diet

Unfortunately, many people in the West tend to take the Ayurvedic diet as synonymous with Indian food. This false notion is created by numerous books on 'Ayurvedic diet' abroad, which simply describe Indian recipes used in modern day India. In fact, these books contain many of the Mogul recipes which are prevalent in north India and have nothing to do in any way with Vedic or Ayurvedic food culture or health in general. Once a participant in my workshop in Austria told me that Ayurvedic cooking was very complicated and not always to the taste of Europeans. She further told me that she tried making Laddoos from a Vedic cookbook and they were awfully sweet. This is a recipe with sugar and fat and in it is neither Ayurvedic nor healthy. In India, there are all kinds of recipes that came from everywhere. It is ridiculous to describe Mogul preparations like this or many others under Ayurvedic or Vedic cooking.

In another incident, one of the student in our Charaka School of Ayurveda who herself was holding workshops on Ayurvedic cooking after having studied for a year in one of the German schools of Ayurveda, did not know about the fundamental qualities of the Ayurvedic food stuffs. I asked her about what was she taught in the German School of Ayurveda. Her reply was very short- 'Italian cooking'. All students had a good laugh at it.

Remember that all Indian foods are not Ayurvedic and Ayurvedic food does not have to be Indian. One can apply Ayurvedic principles of nutrition to any food preparation from any part of the world. Thus, to know the fundamental qualities of food products from the Ayurvedic point of view is extremely essential.

What is Ayurvedic food?

A balanced Ayurvedic food is that which contains all the rasas or tastes and is enriched with herbs and spices to enhance its vitality. A care is taken to eat according to your constitution, season, weather, age and geographical location. The basic qualities of foodstuffs are taken into consideration, as foods are either hot or cold or balanced in their basic nature. Further, there are foods, which are heavy to digest and should be eaten in moderate quantities (see Appendix). The food should be prepared with moderate quantity of fat by altering with plant oils like olive or sesames and animal fat (ghee or clarified butter).

This is a brief description of Ayurvedic food. For details, you can consult my book on this subject. If you are not interested in details, use the recipes or at least their pattern given in this book.

Weekly partial fast

Try and adhere to the routine of a partial fast as described earlier in this book. It gives your system a break and purifies it. The foods described for this particular day are termed as sattvic food in Ayurvedic terminology. Sattva is what brings balance and harmony. This special weekly regimen balances the excesses done with salt, fat or other bulk promoting food like grains during the rest of the week.

Keep vigil

Maintaining weight comprises of keeping a vigil on oneself in diverse manners. It is not done simply by weighing oneself and in case of increase of a few grams, jumping to take drastic measures. You should find the cause and act accordingly. It could be that you put on weight because you ate excessively salty food. Or you ate food with chillies that made you thirsty and your body held water. Or else you ate food that was excessively 'hot' from Ayurvedic point of view and was not balanced with the combination of foods or spices that are 'cold' in nature. That brings too much fire element in the body and one feels more hungry and thirsty. The method to deal with this is to take hot water, tea with some candy sugar in it and some foods which are balanced in nature like carrots, turnips, sweet grapes, sweet apples etc. (see Tables in Appendix).

There could be other situations like eating big and rich meals now and then. Enjoy these great meals but be careful with the quantity. In Ayurveda, it is stated that light meals taken in large quantity are heavy whereas heavy meals consumed in small quantity are light. Make a mental effort to get rid of lobha (greed) of overeating. Excessive eating leads to imbalance of all the energies besides promoting bulk. To strike a balance after a rich meal, you should think of having very simple meal with very little fat for a day two.

For maintaining your weight and proportions of your body, you do not have to weigh and measure or look at the calories every time you eat and drink. This makes life difficult and unpleasant. Live pleasantly, enjoy life but be careful and rational.

Charaka has said very beautifully that the root cause of almost all disorders is *pragyaparadha* or the intellectual error. This error is due to the error in any of the three— knowledge, restraint and memory. Thus, you should apply the knowledge provided in this book to deal with the problem of over-weight. You should exercise restraint from excessive and indiscrete eating and should always remember to do your exercises.

2

Eight Golden Principles of Ayurvedic Nutrition

Most of the time, one has a state of vikriti or imbalance in the body due to wrong food habits. Although I have talked about the essentials of Ayurvedic food culture for building a balance throughout the course of this book, I sum up below the eight essential principles for maintaining weight, equilibrium and health. Therefore strictly follow the principles given below for maintaining balance, right weight and optimum health.

The eight golden principles of Ayurvedic food Culture

Even if the food is prepared by taking care of the rasas and the climate and so on, it can still do harm if the fundamental principles of Ayurvedic food culture are not followed. These are even more important than making the food rejuvenating and balanced.

1. Keep in mind to include all the rasas while **preparing** food. Try to include a variety of ingredients in each meal and take care that you do not eat foods antagonistic in nature (see Appendix for antagonistic foods). Take always warm and fluid food with moderate quantity of fat. Never take preserved foods or those foods which are kept overnight after cooking (*basa*). Food should be **served** in a beautiful manner to create a congenial and aesthetic atmosphere for its consumption.

2. Never **consume** food under stressful circumstances or under any emotional restraint. If you happen to be in such a state shortly before your meal, wait for a while, do some breathing exercises,

wash your face with cold water and then sit comfortably for taking the meal.

3.   **Before beginning your meal**, bring your mind to your food, which is the fundamental basis of body's energy. Look at your food and make a wish that the five elements of the food may provide you with equilibrium, vigour and good health. Say a little prayer or take a few deep breaths.

4.   The food should be **eaten neither too slow nor too fast**. You should not speak with food in your mouth.

5.   Ayurveda recommends **drinking** shortly before meals or one hour after. If required to drink along with food, one may consume liquid in small quantities. Ayurveda recommends drinking only very good quality of wine or beer in a small quantity with food. Juices and milk should not be taken with food. Water is highly recommended but either before or after one hour of eating the meal. Food should be prepared in such a manner that it is fluid and should include some soup or something similar.

6.   Never eat anything **before the previous meal is completely digested.** According to Ayurveda, it is poisonous for the body if one eats when the body is still in the process of digesting the previous meal. Do not eat anything for four hours after having eaten something. For your stomach, a little thing like a piece of chocolate or a fruit is also food to be worked upon and digested. Thus, strictly do not eat anything between meals. If due to some heavy food, you are not hungry for the next meal even after 5 or 6 hours, then avoid taking the meal or take something very light like a soup.

7.   Many people in the world make themselves sick by eating too much. According to Ayurveda, you should always eat so much quantity, which fills the **stomach two third and not completely full**. It means, eat to the limit when you feel comfortably satisfied and not so full that you cannot eat any more. The logic of this is that the

three energies of the body (vata, pitta and kapha) also require place in the stomach for the digestion of the food. If the stomach is made full to its utmost capacity, during digestion, the doshas or energies engaged in digesting the food are pushed out and give rise to vitiation causing various digestive troubles. This may also give rise to *amadosha*. Amadosha is the partial digestion of the food and undigested food remaining in the stomach and intestines, ultimately leads to toxicity in the whole body. For the well-being of the body and for avoiding serious ailments related to digestion, it is absolutely necessary to have discipline about the quantity of food you consume.

8. Never take a **shower** or **bath** immediately after eating. Wait at least two hours, preferably three hours. In any case, it is better to have shower or bath before eating. Also avoid any form of vigorous exercise after food. All these lead to vata vikriti. Going for a slow walk after meals is highly recommended. Dinner should be taken at least two hours before going to bed and you should give a break of about 12 hours at night without any food.

The principles 5, 6 and 7 are extremely important and I have cured many people from their nagging stomach problems by making them follow these. Thus, you should make these eight principles a part of your lifestyle, not only for maintaining your weight but also for safeguarding your health.

3

A Fifteen-minute Yoga Programme

The purpose of doing regular yogic exercises is not to burn the calories but opening the energy channels of the body to keep the body's energies in equilibrium. Yogic movements energise your internal organs and ensure smooth flow of the blood. Give as much importance to do the yogic exercises as you do to brush your teeth or take a shower in the morning. Some people say that they do not have time for it in the morning. Nevertheless, do some stretching exercises in the morning and some yogic exercises in the evening before going to bed. Make sure that you eat your dinner three hours before going to bed so that you are able to do your exercises. In case you are unable to do yogic exercises properly during the week, do for a longer time on the weekend.

Integrate in your routine the simple yogic exercises given in this book. Choose precisely those exercises which you need in your specific case. For example, some of you may have a tendency to put on weight around the waist or abdomen and you can choose exercises specified for this purpose. If you want to learn basics and fundamentals of yoga, refer to my book *Yoga: A Natural Way of Being*.

For maintaining your health, beauty and weight, I suggest that you do *Surya Namaskar* or Prostration to the Sun twelve times every morning. *Surya Namaskar* (SN) exercises your whole body thoroughly. Sun is the symbol of the fire element and as I have stated in the last section of the book, for maintaining weight, the balance of the element fire is extremely important. I do not mean it in an esoteric sense. SN exercises well the place of agni which is the thoracic region of the body, called also the Solar Plexus. Providing exercise to the thoracic region means energising liver, pancreas, gall bladder and stomach. In fact if you have any problem in this region, you will get to know it during these exercises. You may belch if there is some wind trapped in this part; you may feel stiffness or pain in thoracic region signifying hard stomach or some other digestive problem. Thus, the exercises of SN are also an indicator of the state of your agni.

Surya Namaskar or prostration to the sun

Surya Namaskar (SN) involves making 12 different postures one after the other. Either learn the postures one by one gradually from the description given below or learn with a teacher.

1. Face the direction of the sun and stand with folded hands. Your legs should be about 20 cm apart from each other. Put your torso slightly backward and let yourself loose. Close your eyes and concentrate on the image of the sun. You may recite a simple mantra for the sun‾ Om suryayé namah.

2. Slowly raise your folded hands upwards until your head is between your two arms and bend backward in this position. Lean as far back as you comfortably can, making sure that your head is always between your arms.

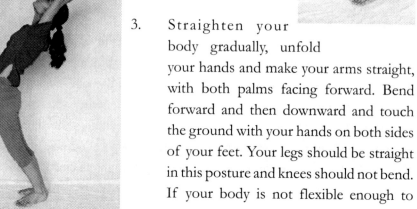

3. Straighten your body gradually, unfold your hands and make your arms straight, with both palms facing forward. Bend forward and then downward and touch the ground with your hands on both sides of your feet. Your legs should be straight in this posture and knees should not bend. If your body is not flexible enough to

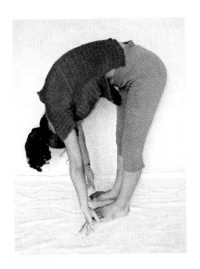

touch the ground, do not force yourself. With repeated practice, you will be able to become flexible.

4. From the above posture, shift your weight to your hands and your left leg and stretch the right leg backwards so that it rests on the knee and the front part of your foot. In this process, your left leg is folded. Bend your head backward.

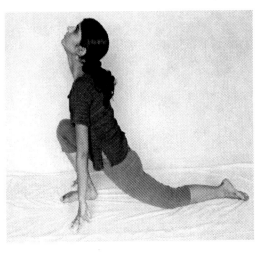

5. Bring your bent head forward and shift your body weight to both your hands. Stretch back the right leg. Make a straight line with your body by shifting your

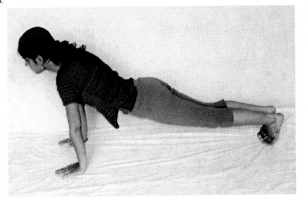

Your hands. Stretch back the right leg. Make a straight line with your body by shifting your weight to your hands and toes. Your head should be in line with the rest of your body.

6.   In position 5, you are touching the ground with four parts of your body. This position is made by touching the ground with eight parts of the body and that is why it is called Ashatanaga Pranama (prostration with eight parts of the body). In addition to your hands and feet, touch the ground with both your knees, chest and forehead. Your stomach and thighs should not touch the ground.

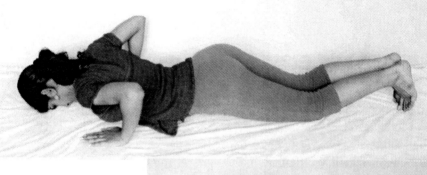

7.   Put your weight on your hands and feet and gradually raise your head. Bend your head backward as far as you comfortably can.

8.   Slowly bring your head forwards from the previous position, raise your body in the middle while putting your weight on your hands and feet.

Your head should remain between your arms, while your feet should be in a flat position with soles touching the ground.

9. Bring the right leg forward, stretch back the left leg, put your weight on your hands and make your arms straight. Bend your head backward. This position is the same as position 4 except that here the right leg is forward instead of the left leg.

10. This position is the same the as Position 3. From position 9, bring your stretched leg forward and put this foot parallel to the other foot between your two hands. In this process, your body will be slightly lifted. Keep your legs straight and do not bend your knees.

11. Straighten your body from the previous position and raise your arms upward; fold your hands and bend backward as you did in Position 2.

12. This is the last position and here you come back to Position 1, from where you started.

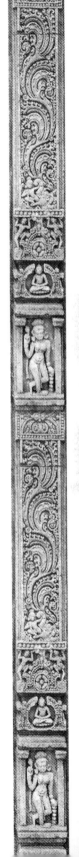

4

Avoiding Weight-enhancing Factors

This is an obvious reminder to control weight and I need not repeat anything which has been already said in this book. Once you have succeeded in balancing your weight and to trim your body at the right places, you should very carefully and consciously avoid the weight-enhancing factor described earlier in order to maintain weight. Go back to Chapter 1 of Section I of the book and recall all those causative factors that make you gain extra bulk and upset the shape of your body. This is the primary level of working towards weight control. If you are doing other things like exercises and walks and are careless about other fundamental weight-enhancing factors, it is like adding fuel to the fire with one hand and adding water to extinguish it with the other hand.

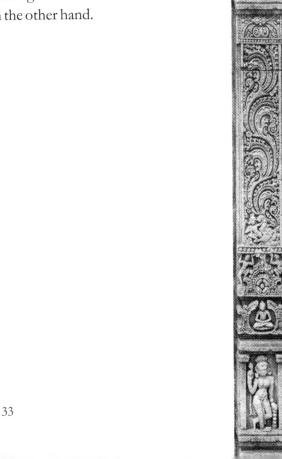

5

Taking Weight-Reducing Remedies

Normally if you follow the instructions in previous four chapters, you probably would not need to take the weight-reducing remedies (See Section I, Chapter 5). However, there can be unavoidable circumstances in your life that may lead to gain weight. I am giving below some situations where people fall prey to gain weight. The wise thing is not to fall into the vicious cycle again and act immediately by taking one of the remedies for a few days and then follow other instructions to maintain weight.

Special situations for taking weight-reducing remedies

I give below some special circumstances that cause to gain weight and the remedies suggested in each specific case.

☐   Sometimes one gains weight due to temporary disability that forces a sedentary lifestyle. For example, a broken bone or a ligament or something alike can bring a stop to the usual activities of life. Nevertheless, one should try to move the individual body parts in these circumstances and should eat nourishing but controlled diet. However, if you end up gaining some kilos or gather flesh at undesired places, take care immediately. Make sure that you do not let your temporary forced sedentary lifestyle become your habit. Sometimes, the extra weight gives a person inertia and that leads to gain even more weight. As it is, a person is fatigued due to an accident or injury and tends to fall prey to the inactive lifestyle and lethargy. In these circumstances, I suggest that you take Trifala treatment in honey for two weeks. This will help you gain energy, lose weight and make you feel active. Trifala is a rasayana (vitalising substance), as well and it will give you vitality.

☐ Many people gain weight due to an imbalance caused by the intake of allopathic drugs. Their body starts holding water and the agni gets disturbed. They begin to eat a lot and consume excessive quantity of liquids. The remedy in this case is also Trifala but take it with water after soaking it overnight. After you have finished the allopathic treatment, take Trifala regularly for three weeks. It will purify your body, re-establish the balance of three energies (vata, pitta and kapha), and will revitalise you. It will help you throw out the impurities and will save you from the long-term side-effects of the drugs.

☐ Too many festivals and too many parties in a short span of time may lead you to put on weight. Many people go for organised holiday tours which offer several big meals a day. In fact, these tours allure people with this offer of three major meals and an afternoon tea and a cake. Most people cherish all what they can eat thinking that they have paid for it. In fact, they lose their restraint and end up gaining weight and getting disturbed agni. The remedy for this is to refrain from booking such holidays. The second remedy is to control your mind and divert it to health remembering the following─ 'All that what is good, excess of it is bad'. If it is already too late and you find yourself with some extra hanging flesh around your waist or get a paunch, take purgation once a week for four weeks and take diet described in Section I, Chapter 2.

Appendix

Description of Some Terms and Products Mentioned in the Book

Ayurvedic qualities of some basic foods

During the course of this book, I have mentioned about the fundamental nature of various food products. You need to take care not to prepare food with extreme cold and extreme hot products. Their combination makes them balanced.

Besides the fundamental nature of various food products, you have to pay attention to the foods which are heavy to digest (Table 4). You should eat them in small quantities and make balanced preparations to accompany them or make them balanced by adding balanced herbs and spices and agni-promoting spices like pepper, ajwain and cumin.

The fifth and the last table gives you a list of products which are antagonistic in combination with each other, and you should avoid them. They slowly poison the body and make you sick.

I suggest that you make a copy of these tables and hang in your kitchen. By regular practice, you will ultimately remember the basic quality of the food products.

-----------------------------------Table 1-----------------------------------
FOODS COLD IN NATURE

Grains: Wheat, rice, maize (promotes vata), barley (increases vata), common millet and Italian millet (enhances vata), masoor beans (also called red lentils) (promotes vata), young green peas, ripe green peas (strongly vata promoting), chick peas

Vegetables: Spinach, cabbage and Brussels sprouts (vata), okra, green beans, bitter gourd, endives, fennel, aubergine, onion, celery, cucumber, beetroot, sweet paprika (without seeds), dandelion, asparagus

Fruit: Apples (sweet), bananas, pears, apricot, guava, muskmelon, water melon, figs

Dairy products: Milk, ghee, butter

Meat: Frog, seafood, sea fish, mutton

Herbs and spices: Clove, coriander, fennel, anise, dill leaves (not the seeds), liquorice

Others: Sugar

-------------------------------------Table 2-------------------------------------
FOODS HOT IN NATURE

Grains: Urad beans, soya beans

Vegetables: cress salad, potatoes, cauliflower, tomatoes

Fruit: Oranges, grapefruit, lemon, grapes (which are not absolutely sweet), peaches, plumbs, kiwis (specially the black seeds in kiwi), nuts (almonds, peanuts, hazelnuts, walnuts, pine nuts and others), sour apples

Dairy products: Yoghurt, processed cheese

Meat: Pork, horse, beef, freshwater fish

Herbs and spices: Greater or large cardamom, cumin, cinnamon, black pepper or white pepper, fenugreek, kalonji, garlic, basil, dill seeds, ajwain, mustard seeds, nutmeg, mint

Others: Honey, vegetable oils, eggs (hen, fish)

--Table 3--
FOODS WITH NATURAL EQUILIBRIUM

Grains: Finger millet, mung beans, chickpeas at the beginning of germination

Vegetables: Carrots, turnips, small radishes (not over-ripe), zucchini, pumpkin (just ripened),

Fruit: Sweet mangoes, papaya, pomegranate, grapes (sweet)

Meat: Deer, goat, chicken

Herbs and spices: Small cardamom, ginger, Turmeric or curcuma

--Table 4--
HEAVY TO DIGEST FOODS

Vegetarian foods: Urad beans, over-ripe peas, animal or plant fat, nuts or preparation from nuts, any vegetable or fruit or a preparation of food that has an extreme taste like sour, sweet, pungent, bitter, astringent, salty and when consumed in excess, raw or over-ripe vegetables and fruits, yoghurt when eaten several times a day and specially at night

Non-vegetarian foods: Pork, beef, meat of animals kept under stressful conditions, animal fat or foods containing animal fat in larger quantities.

--Table 5--
ANTAGONISTIC FOOD COMBINATIONS
----

1. Milk in combination with sour foods, radish, water melon or fish
2. Honey in any heated form or taking a hot drink immediately after taking honey
3. Fatty food in combination with cold drinks or cold water
4. Use of diet adverse to a person's food habits
5. Intake of food stuffs which are hot and cold in temperature at the same time.

6.   Food antagonism to time, place and constitution

7.   Foods excessively dominating in one particular rasa like excessively salty, sweet, sour etc.

Bulk-promoting foods

Grains and lentils: Most grains are bulk promoting with the exception of barley. In particular, maize and chickpea flour (Besan) are highly bulk promoting. Massor and Mung beans are least bulk-enhancing out of all the lentils and beans. Flour made from the roasted wheat grains is not bulk promoting.

Fruits: Bananas

Meats: Most meets except deer, goat, birds and seafood are bulk promoting. Pork is highly bulk promoting.

Dairy products: All dairy products except buttermilk are bulk-promoting. Yoghurt, cream, butter and ghee are highly bulk-promoting.

Others: Oils, plant fat, animal fat, nuts, alcoholic beverages, too much salt, too much sugar containing things like chocolates and other sweet stuff, all kinds of fried stuff are bulk promoting.

Bulk-reducing foods

Grains: Barley is bulk reducing. In general, roasted grains are bulk-decreasing. Thus, if you are fond of bread, roast the wheat or other grains and then make flour for the bread. Similarly, roasted black chickpeas, which are used to make sattu are bulk-decreasing.

Fruits and vegetables: Most fruits and vegetables are bulk decreasing. In particular, green vegetables are bulk-reducing. Use of the balanced vegetables and fruits given in the tables above is highly recommended. Papaya and pear are in particular bulk-decreasing and their use is highly recommended.

Dairy products: Buttermilk is bulk-decreasing.

Herbs and spices: Ginger, dried ginger called shunthi, black pepper, Long pepper, curcuma, cumin, dill seeds, Ajwain, thyme, mint, kalonji are bulk decreasing because of their effect on agni. Normally, all the other spices and herbs generally used for cooking are also bulk decreasing.

Others: Hot water, water with lemon and honey*.

Description of some spices

Most spices described in this book are quite common and generally people in the West know about them. I am describing below some spices that are not so well known so that you have facility to find them after obtaining knowledge about them. The best source to obtain the good quality spices abroad is the Indian or oriental shops. Even if they do not have certain things, they can order them for you. There are certain other things you can get at the organic seed shops.

Long pepper (Piper longum)

It is called pippalli in Sanskrit and peepal in Hindi. There are two varieties available. One is small and thin, about 1-2 centimetres (0.4 to 0.8 inch) long and ½ cm (0.2 inch) in diameter. The second variety is double the size than this. Long pepper has a granular surface. From the surface, both the varieties look alike. Long pepper is less hot in its Ayurvedic properties than the normal black pepper. It is recommended to use it in spice mixtures and some teas. It is very good for the nerves. It has weight decreasing qualities because of its effect on agni.

Kalonji (Nigella sativa)

Outside India, kalonji is called by several erroneous names like black cumin or small fennel or onion seeds, etc. One should be very careful in

---

* Honey should never be used in hot water. However, you can use warm water. Honey heated above 40^0C is toxic.

buying it and make sure that the word 'kalonji' is written on the packet. Its Latin name is *Nigella sativa* and popular name in some southern countries is Nigella. It is originally from southern Europe but now a very important Indian spice, which is cultivated all over India.

Kalonji is hot in its Ayurvedic nature. It has a strong taste and flavour and therefore it should not be used in delicately flavoured dishes.

Ajwain

Seeds of Ajwain which are used as spice are tiny, dull brown with lines on the surface. Ajwain is two kinds— big and small. Small is 1-2 mm (about 1/20 of an inch) and the big one is double its size. In India, big one is generally given to house animals for various remedies and small one is used as spice and in medicines.

Ajwain is similar to thyme in properties. However, thyme leaves are used whereas seeds are used in case of ajwain. Ajwain is profusely used in food and medicine in India and is cultivated almost everywhere. It is hot in its Ayurvedic nature.

It cures aggravated vata and kapha and enhances pitta. It promotes digestion and is extremely effective to cure several digestive disorders. It gives a delicious taste and flavour to various food preparations. Ajwain promotes the liver function and hence helps digest heavy and rich foods. To balance agni, take Ajwain along with ginger and rock salt.

Dill (Soye in Hindi)

It is a common herb in the West but in the present context, dill seeds are used. Dill leaves are cold in their Ayurvedic nature whereas seeds are extremely hot. Dill leaves are eaten as herb or vegetable and seeds are used as spice and medicine. Dill seeds are important for women and are used in many remedies to cure menstrual troubles and for the management of post-delivery period.

Dill Seeds render delicious taste and flavour to food. Since they are highly pitta promoting, they should not be used excessively, or with foods which are hot in nature. They should be avoided in hot climate. To neutralise the hot effect of dill, you may use it in combination with fennel seeds.

Cress (Chansur or Halim in Hindi)

Seeds are round and are brown in colour. They are very strong as spice and they are mostly used in several remedies. Cress seeds are blood purifier. As you all know, the small, rounded leaves of cress are delicious as salad. In India, the leaves are principally used as fodder for horses, camels and other house animals. Because of their tremendous medicinal value, I suggest that cress seeds should be used to garnish various salads or they can be put directly in different dough preparations or in sandwiches and so on.

Cress is hot in its Ayurvedic nature. Leaves are mild hot because of the bitter rasa in them but seeds are extremely hot. Germination makes them milder.

Saffron (Kesar in Hindi)

Saffron is like tiny fibres of bright red and orange colour. These fibres are stamina of the delicate flowers of *Crocus sativus*. The saffron plant is originally from southern Europe. It is cultivated in Spain, Italy, Greece and France and exported from there to many parts of the world. In India, it is cultivated in Jammu and Kashmir and is also imported from France and Spain.

When taken in small quantities and regularly, saffron helps bring the equilibrium of the three doshas. Basically, its Ayurvedic nature is hot and it should not be taken more than 250 milligrams daily. It is an aphrodisiac and a rasayana.*

---

* See my books *The Kamasutra for Women* and *Companionship and Sexuality* for the recipes of aphrodisiacs with saffron.

Holy Basil (Tulsi in Hindi)

This plant is originally from India. It is called Holy basil or *Oscimum sanctum* in Latin because it is worshipped in every Hindu home. Because of its tremendous medicinal qualities, perhaps the sages made all these rituals for the care and protection of this plant and ensured its ready availability in every home.

Basil leaves make the food rejuvenating. One should regularly use basil in the form of tea or to flavour the salads. It is a rasayana and strengthens the immune system. It is hot in its Ayurvedic nature and therefore should not be used in excess. The daily dose is four to five leaves. The European variety of Basil with big leaves is milder and may be taken double this quantity.

Fenugreek (Methi in Hindi)

Fenugreek seeds are used as spice and for medicinal purposes and leaves are eaten as vegetable. Fenugreek is hot in its Ayurvedic nature and seeds have a very strong taste. This spice is not used in delicately flavoured dishes. It is very good for curing vitiated vata and is highly recommended when one gradually steps into middle age.

Salts

Most people in the world know about sea salt, which is widely used. From Ayurvedic point of view, there are four kinds of other salts. For the purpose of cooking, there are two kinds of rock salts which are important besides the generally available sea salt.

Sendhav or *Sendha* salt is transparent rock salt, which has shades of other colours in it as it is enriched with other minerals. It is being marketed as Himalayan salt in Europe these days.

Krishan lavan or *kala namak* or black salt is generally dark brown because it contains iron and sulphur.

For everyday use mix different kinds of salts in equal quantity with water in a glass jar and use this concentrated salted water while cooking.

AUM SHANTI

About the author

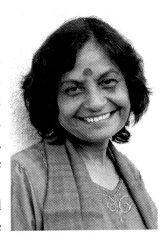

After a doctorate degree in reproduction biology in India, Dr. Verma studied Neurobiology in Paris University and obtained a second doctorate. She pursued advanced research at the National Institutes of Health, Bethesda (USA) and the Max-Planck Institute in Freiburg, Germany. At the peak of her career in medical research in a pharmaceutical company in Germany, she realised that the modern approach to health care is basically fragmented and non-holistic. Besides, we are directing all our efforts and resources to cure disease rather than maintaining health. In response, Dr. Verma founded NOW in 1986 to spread the message of holistic living, preventive methods for health care and to promote the use of mild medicine and various self-help therapeutic measures.

Dr. Verma grew up with a strong familial tradition of Ayurveda with a grandmother who had enormous Ayurvedic wisdom and was a gifted healer. She has been studying Ayurveda in the traditional Guru-shishya style with Acharya Priya Vrat Sharma of the Benares Hindu University for the last 21 years and completed her doctorate.

Dr. Verma is an ardent researcher and is working hard to compile the living tradition of Ayurveda and spread it in the world through her books. She has published over eighteen books on yoga, Ayurveda, women and Companionship. The books are published in various languages of the world. Besides, she has published numerous scientific papers. Several other books are in preparation. She lectures extensively, teaches in Europe for several months a year, trains students at her two centres in India and gives radio and television programmes. Her film on Ayurveda was shown in 100 countries in 130 languages.

Dr. Verma has founded Charaka School of Ayurveda to train interested people with genuine Ayurvedic education so that they can further impart the knowledge of Ayurvedic way of life and save people from becoming a victim of charlatanry in Ayurveda.

Dr. Verma is doing several research projects on medicinal plants and their combination in the form of remedies. She has also taken up a social service project to distribute and promote the use of Ayurvedic remedies and yoga therapy in rural areas of India. She does regular lectures for school children in the rural and remote areas of the Himalayas to promote wisdom of traditional science and medicine.

Dr. Verma gives seminars, lectures and teaches in the Charaka School of Ayurveda with guru-shishya tradition. She is the Academic Director of the Charaka Ayurveda and Yoga Academy and Cultural Centre (CAYACC), which has its headquarters in Dresden. She is a visiting professor in Beirat des Berufsverbandes Unabhängiger Gesundheitswissenschaftlicher Yoga-LehrerInnen (BUGY) in Göttingen (Germany).

Dr Verma speaks Hindi, Punjabi, French, German and English and she has knowledge of Sanskrit.

Author's Publications

1. *Patanjali's Yoga Sutra: A Scientific Exposition* (Published in English, Hindi and German).

2. *Ayurveda for Inner Harmony: Nutrition, Sexual Energy and Healing* (Published in English, German, Italian, French, Romanian and Hindi).

3. *Ayurveda a Way of Life* (Published in English, German, Italian, French, Spanish, Czech, Greek, Portuguese and Hindi).

4. *The Kamasutra for Women* (Published in English [America and India], German, French, Dutch, Romanian, Italian, Portuguese, Hindi and Malayalam).

5. *Stress-free Work with Yoga and Ayurveda* (Published in German, English [America and India] and Hindi).

6. *Patanjali and Ayurvedic Yoga* (Published in English, German and Hindi).

7. *Programming Your Life with Ayurveda* (Published in German, French and English).

8. *Ayurvedic Food Culture and Recipes* (Published in English, German and Hindi).

9. *Yoga: A Natural Way of Being* (Published in English, German, French, Italian and Hindi).

10. *Companionship and Sexuality (Based on Ayurveda and the Hindu tradition)* (Published in English and German).

11. *Natural Glamour: The Ayurveda Beauty Book* (Published in German and English)

12. *Losing and Maintaining Weight with Ayurveda and Yoga* (Published in English and German).

13. *The Timeless Wisdom of Ayurveda: A Scientific Exposition* (in press)

14. *Prakriti and Pulse: The Two Mysteries of Ayurveda* (in press)

15. *Good Food for Dogs: Vegetarian nourishment based on Ayurvedic wisdom* (in

press)

16. *Diet for Losing Weight* (in press)

17. *Aum: The Infinite Energy* (in press)

18. *Bala Kamasutra: Aphorisms for Imparting Sexual education to Children* (in preparation)

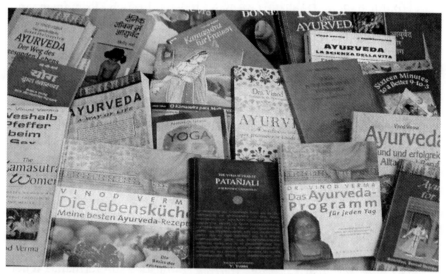

For more information about the books and the publication rights, contact the author at ayurvedavv@yahoo.com or drvinodverma@dataone.in

The Charaka School of Ayurveda and Patanjali Yogadarshana Society

(Himalayan Centre)

The Charka School of Ayurveda (CSA) has been founded by Dr. Vinod Verma to spread the genuine classical tradition as well as the living tradition of Ayurveda in the world for promoting healthy living and preventing ailments. Its aim is to teach people a healthy lifestyle which enhances immunity and vitality and enables them to live a life with optimum level of energy. For minor ailments, people should be capable of using home remedies, appropriate physical and mental exercises and nutrition.

CSA aims to bring genuine and practical aspects of Ayurveda to people and save them from Americanised and Europeanised distorted versions of Ayurveda and other forms of charlatanry that do more harm than good.

To achieve this purpose, CSA organises to train students in Europe who can further spread the message of Ayurvedic lifestyle and help people with genuine massages, purification practices, nutrition and other practical aspects of Ayurveda. The school is in association with the most learned persons of Ayurveda in India and several exclusive persons involved in health education in Europe.

The object of Patanjali Yogadarshana Society is to spread the message of Patanjali in the world. The wisdom of the Yoga Sutras is not only beneficial for the yogis but also for our day-to-day normal life. Its aim is to enhance *sattva* or the inner stillness and peace in the world as well as in the individual minds. With years of research on Yoga and Ayurveda, Dr. Verma has founded the Ayurvedic Yoga and has written a book on the subject.

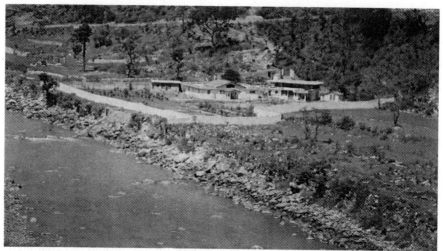

Himalayan Centre

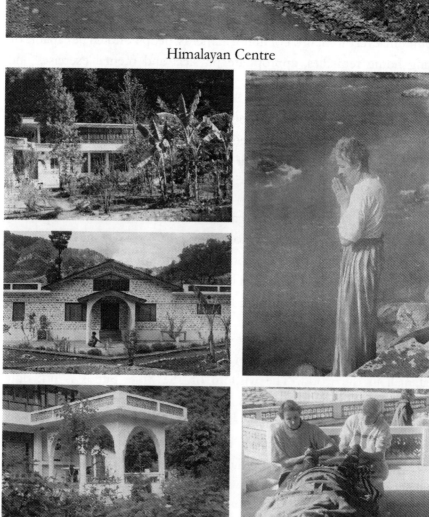

Lectures, Seminars and Training Programmes

To get detailed information on the Charaka School of Ayurveda as well as our other programmes in India and Europe, visit our website or write to the following addresses:

The New Way Health Organisation .NOW.

A-130, Sector 26, Noida 201301, U.P., India

Tel. 0091 (0)120 2527820 or (0)9412224820

Email: ayurvedavv@yahoo.com or drvinodverma@dataone.in

Website: www.ayurvedavv.com

Contacts in Europe:

In Germany:

Michael Röslen

Berufsverband Unabhängiger Gesundheitswissenschaftlicher Yoga LehrerInnen (BUGY)

Tel/Fax: 0049 (0) 5508 92135 Email: bugyoga@t-online.de

In Switzerland:

Gisela Binder, Tel. 0041 61 (0) 6923849, Fax: -6923502

Charaka Ayurvedic Products (CAP) -- A sub-unit of NOW

Due to the increasing popularity of Ayurveda all over the world, a demand for its products has increased. We specially focus at supplying products Dr. Vinod Verma has mentioned in her books. But we can supply you any product that belongs to the original Ayurvedic Himalayan tradition. Our products are made under Dr. Verma's guidance. Our motto is to maintain quality at all costs.

Our production unit is located in our pollution-free Himalayan Centre with home grown products. For more details of bulk, retail and e-mail orders of products, contact: ayurvedavv@yahoo.com

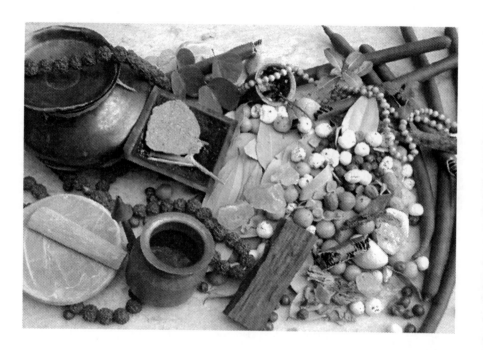